Decision Making in Aesthetic Practice

Decision Making in Aesthetic Practice

The Right Procedures for the Right Patients

Edited by

VINCENT WONG, BSc, MBChB
VINDOC AESTHETICS
LONDON, UK

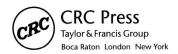

CRC Press
Taylor & Francis Group
Boca Raton London New York

CRC Press is an imprint of the
Taylor & Francis Group, an **informa** business

First edition published 2022
by CRC Press

2 Park Square, Milton Park, Abingdon, Oxon, OX14 4RN

and by CRC Press

6000 Broken Sound Parkway NW, Suite 300, Boca Raton, FL 33487-2742

© 2022 Taylor & Francis Group, LLC

CRC Press is an imprint of Taylor & Francis Group, LLC

Library of Congress Cataloging-in-Publication Data

Names: Wong, Vincent (Cosmetic doctor), editor.
Title: Decision making in aesthetic practice : the right procedures for the right patients / edited by Vincent Wong.
Description: First edition. | Boca Raton : CRC Press, 2022. | Includes bibliographical references and index. | Summary: "Healthcare professionals in Aesthetic Practice are often faced with a presenting complaint that may seem straightforward to treat but lends itself to more than one treatment option. The aim of this book is to help guide a healthcare professional in selecting the best and most appropriate options for any patient"-- Provided by publisher.
Identifiers: LCCN 2021011775 (print) | LCCN 2021011776 (ebook) | ISBN 9781032046037 (hardback) | ISBN 9780367769802 (paperback) | ISBN 9781003193883 (ebook)
Subjects: MESH: Cosmetic Techniques | Reconstructive Surgical Procedures | Clinical Decision-Making | Esthetics | Patient-Centered Care
Classification: LCC RD119 (print) | LCC RD119 (ebook) | NLM WO 595 | DDC 617.9/5--dc23
LC record available at https://lccn.loc.gov/2021011775
LC ebook record available at https://lccn.loc.gov/2021011776

ISBN: 978-1-032-04603-7 (hbk)
ISBN: 978-0-367-76980-2 (pbk)
ISBN: 978-1-003-19388-3 (ebk)

Typeset in Times
by KnowledgeWorks Global Ltd.

Contents

Preface

The creation of this book stemmed from my passion for Medical Aesthetics – not just the practice of it, but also teaching and developing new and better treatment protocols for our patients.

Healthcare professionals in our speciality are often faced with a presenting complaint that may seem straightforward to treat but lend itself to more than one treatment option. To achieve and deliver natural-looking results, certain proportions of the face must be respected, as well as having a good understanding of the root cause of the complaint and sharing that knowledge with patients. This book has been structured in such a way that we can focus on one area of the face in turn, to help readers gain insight into that specific anatomical region.

In a booming and ever-expanding industry, it is crucial that healthcare professionals have a good understanding of various treatment modalities. From my personal experience, I find that combinations of various types of treatments often work better than a stand-alone treatment. Hence, it is a great pleasure to be able to share my experience and suggestions in various sections of this book.

As facial aesthetics has multiple facets, I would not have been able to provide a comprehensive overview without having the honour to have contributions from several esteemed co-authors of various backgrounds. To provide the best care for our patients, we must understand the limitations of Medical Aesthetics; some patients are better suited for surgical procedures and I am glad that we have been able to include the synergy and differences between surgical and non-surgical approaches to facial aesthetics.

Facial aesthetics has progressed from 'wrinkle chasing' to a more holistic approach. In these modern times, our speciality is no longer aimed at mature women as it once was. Furthermore, I am proud to be able to celebrate the diversity in this book by including case studies of patients of different ages, ethnicities, genders, and sexualities.

The aim of this book is to help and guide healthcare professionals in making the best and most appropriate decisions for their patients. I hope that you find this book useful in helping you select the right treatments for the right patients in your own practice.

Vincent Wong

Acknowledgements

The publishers are very grateful to Primal Pictures for permission to adapt several images from www.anatomy.tv. The authors would also like to credit Frederick Wong for the images and illustrations.

Contributors

Sue Ann Chan
Consultant Dermatologist
Skin Clinic Victoria Street
    and Harley Street
King's College Hospital NHS
    Foundation Trust
Beckenham Beacon
London, UK
and
Princess Royal University Hospitals
Orpington, UK

Darika de Bacq Rose
Aesthetic Doctor
Dr Rose Club
Wirral, UK

Adnan Erdem
Plastic, Reconstructive
    and Aesthetic Surgeon
Private Practice
Bursa, Turkey

Chris Gill
Aesthetics Business Consultant
Allergan Aesthetics
London, UK

Kelly Morrell
Hair Restoration Consultant & Scalp
    Micropigmentation Technician
The Private Clinic of Harley Street
London, UK

Naomi O'Hara Collins
Scalp Micropigmentation Technician
Naomi O'Hara Permanent Cosmetics
Portsmouth, UK

Alexander Parys
Aesthetic Doctor
Dr Alexander James Aesthetics
Manchester, UK

Mehmet Veli Karaaltin
Professor of Plastic, Aesthetic
    and Reconstructive Surgery
Karaaltın Plastic Surgery Clinic
Istanbul, Turkey

Sarah Whitehead
Aesthetic Nurse
SW Aesthetics Training Ltd
Ashbourne, UK

Frederick Wong
Digital Graphics and Creative Designer
Johor Bahru, Malaysia

Vincent Wong
Cosmetic Doctor
VINDOC Aesthetics
London, UK

1

The Cosmetic Consultation

Chris Gill and Vincent Wong

CONTENTS

You never get a second chance to make a first impression

The cosmetic consultation is the key step in building a good rapport with your patient. It is your opportunity to understand what your patients want, what brought them to your service, and how you can help them with their needs. There are three key points to remember in a successful cosmetic consultation:

- How well the healthcare provider listens to the patient's concerns.
- How well the healthcare provider explains the treatment options.
- How well the healthcare provider answers the questions from the patient.

Consultation methods have evolved over the years in medical aesthetics and now take two distinct paths.

The first method is offering a 'transactional consultation', out of necessity, because it is required. This allows the healthcare provider time to complete the necessary paperwork before the treatment can go ahead. They often find that the patient leads these types of consultation. The patient already has an idea of what treatment they would like and what their budget is going to be. Essentially, the patient is self-diagnosing and then telling the practitioner what their treatment should be. This is not ideal – this underwhelming form of consultation generally takes 20–30 minutes, at most, and on some occasions is immediately followed up by a treatment. The consultation will be booked out for a specific treatment, e.g. dermal fillers, and this will then set the precedent that the consultation will focus on that certain treatment and what it can offer. It doesn't leave room for educating patients about all the treatment options available to them. However, it can be an efficient business/consultation model as it allows you to financially benefit from a consultation, and it provides the patient with a treatment during the same visit. Most healthcare providers at the start of their medical aesthetics career will begin with this model, and some will never change.

The other type of consultation is 'patient-centric' and is focused on understanding patient needs and educating them so they have a better understanding of why certain conditions or concerns appear on their bodies. The healthcare provider will control the consultation and recommend a treatment or treatment plan that they believe will deliver the best results for the patient, based on their needs, rather than focusing on the treatment the patient had predetermined that they wanted before the consultation. These consultations can last up to 60 minutes and generally then encourage the patient to rebook for their treatment later. It will focus on the patient; it will not be treatment specific, and it will set the tone for the relationship going forward. It will be the most important part of the patient's treatment journey. Remember that a patient's budget at their first visit can be very different at their second visit, especially when faced with a bespoke treatment plan that exceeds the patient's expectations. This is an added value consultation where the healthcare provider seeks to educate the patient, impart their knowledge, and provide a patient-centric treatment plan.

An example of how a patient-centric consultation can benefit both the patients and the business is as follows. An existing patient is sitting in the waiting room and is discussing their prior first treatment with a new patient. They were complimentary about the treatment, but they couldn't speak highly enough about the consultation and what they had learnt. Then imagine the existing patient said the following sentence 'you will never have had a consultation like this before'. In an industry where word of mouth is key to success, imagine what you could achieve if every patient you consulted said a similar message to their family and friends?

When Does the Consultation Start?

It is not always obvious, but a consultation starts when the patient walks through the door for the first time. There are, however, a few important tricks of the trade to consider before they do.

A website is your virtual receptionist. It allows you to deliver an exact message to your patients consistently, time and time again. The same applies to social media, digital advertising, and in fact any type of platform in which you control the content. These are ideal places to start educating your potential patient on what to expect in your consultation. You will hear the phrase 'managing their expectations' a lot in medical aesthetics and this is where you start to do that.

The most likely next step is that the potential patient will look to book a consultation. This can be offered in so many ways these days, but no matter which way an appointment is booked it still presents an opportunity to educate patients. Having a text message, voice message, email, etc. explaining how you work and what they are to expect will help set the tone for when the patient walks through your door.

Before you see the patient, it is most likely that they will be greeted by someone else upon their arrival. Whether this is a positive or negative experience, it will have a significant impact on the mentality of the patient when they enter the room. Make sure this experience is above their expectations; it is important to always greet people with eye contact, a smile, and a positive tone. This will always be well received, even if they don't show it. Ask whoever greets the patient to provide clear instructions as to what is to happen before the consultation, whether it be where to sit, medical forms to read, or a treatment questionnaire to complete. It is important that the patient feels welcomed and looked after.

The above may seem simple but a challenge to yourself would be to deliver this well on a consistent basis. If you succeed, your patient will always be educated and positive when they enter the room.

What Can I Do to Make My Consultation Effective?

Asking patients to complete a treatment questionnaire before the consultation will allow them to formulate and communicate their interests and provide you with a better understanding of what the patient desires. There are many versions of these questionnaires (see, e.g. Figure 1.1); however, the most important part is making sure that it is positioned to the patient as an important part of the consultation and not just a selling tool. If the patient sees value in completing it, then the information will be beneficial to the consultation. (See further below on key performance indicators [KPIs].)

The consultation process should include the following steps:

- *Assessment:* This is where the healthcare professional assesses the patient's health and motivations and provides expert opinion. Assessing the patient's motivations and aspirations will help you formulate the patient's needs, which is often misaligned. For example, a patient with thin and sun-damaged skin requests a thread lift procedure to reduce the appearance of wrinkles; however, the patient may need other treatments to improve the quality of the skin first, in order for any subsequent procedures to be successful.

Aesthetic Interest Questionnaire

Date: _____

Patient name: _____

Date of birth: _____

What is the main reason for your visit today?

_____

_____

_____

_____

_____

I would like to be advised on:

☐ How I can look better for my age

☐ How I can change something that
has been bothering me for years

☐ How I can look more attractive

☐ Other: _____

_____

Have you had a consultation or treatment
for a cosmetic procedure before?

☐ Yes   ☐ No

How often do you think about wanting
a cosmetic procedure?

☐ Most days   ☐ Weekly   ☐ Monthly

Which three statements
best reflect how you would
like to look and feel after
the treatment?

☐ I want to look less tired   ☐ I want a less saggy appearance   ☐ I want my face to look slimmer

☐ I want to look less angry   ☐ I want to look more youthful   ☐ I want softer features

☐ I want to look less sad   ☐ I want to look more attractive

Please circle the area(s) of your interest:

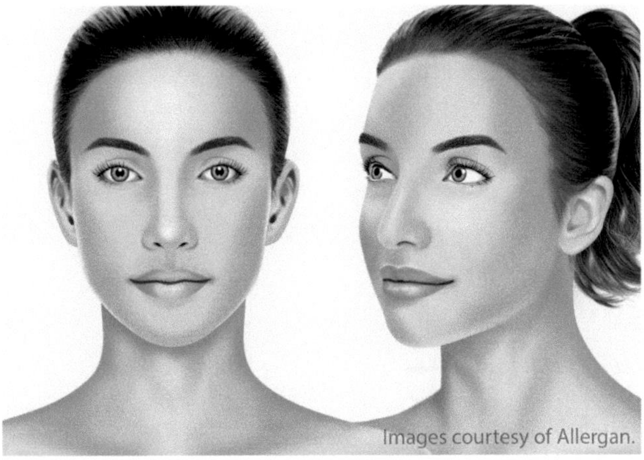

Images courtesy of Allergan.

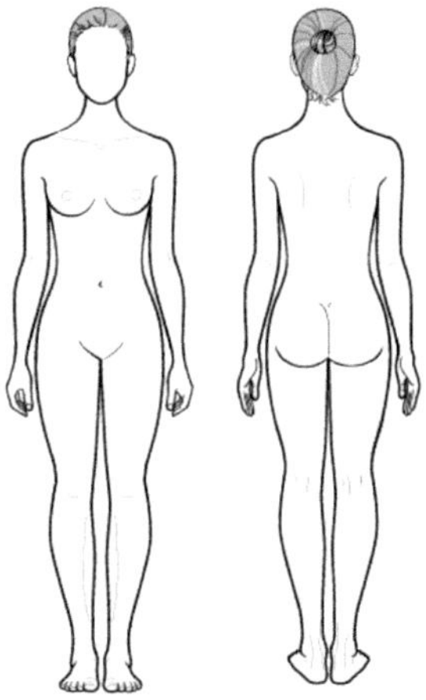

FIGURE 1.1 Aesthetic interest questionnaire. (©2021 Allergan; used with permission; all rights reserved.)

(Continued)

How would you rate the quality of your skin?   Poor   Fair   Good   Very Good   Excellent
(Please circle the appropriate answer)

                                                                      Hydration   Elasticity   Smoothness   Color

If you could enhance an aspect of your skin,
what would you enhance?
(Please circle the appropriate answer)

These treatments/products interest me:
(Please circle the treatment area(s) that interest you)

SKIN ENHANCEMENT	FACIAL IMPROVEMENT	BODY CONTOURING	OTHER
Skin injectables	Facial fillers	Fat reduction	Laser hair removal
Skin products	Wrinkle relaxers	Breast enlargement	Hair replacement
Laser treatment	Face lifting	Breast correction	Waxing
Peeling	Ear correction	Tummy tuck	Labiaplasty
Microdermabrasion	Fat reduction – chin	Arm lift	Scar revision
Facial	Nose surgery	Buttock augmentation	
Skin tightening	Eyelid correction		
	Brow correction		

How did you hear about us?

☐ My doctor   ☐ Search engine
☐ My insurance company   ☐ Social media platform
   provider   ☐ Seminar
☐ Advertisements/periodicals   ☐ Other
☐ A friend or family member

Contact information

☐ I would like to receive information about
   new products/trends/our clinic

☐ You are allowed to contact me for further
   questions concerning an appointment at
   your clinic

Phone number: _____

E-mail address: _____

Signature: _____

Prepared by Allergan, January 2017, INT/0318/2016(1)

FIGURE 1.1   Aesthetic interest questionnaire. *(Continued)*

- *Root cause education:* This is where the healthcare professional educates the patient on skin and facial anatomy, including the effects of chronological ageing on skin, fat, muscles, and bone. This will help patients understand the concerns they see in the mirror.
- *Providing treatment options:* This is an opportunity for the healthcare professional to present specific treatment options (based on the first two steps), which will meet both the patient's wants and needs.
- *Treatment education:* After presenting treatment options, the healthcare professional should educate the patient on the specific details of the proposed treatments (e.g. mechanism of action, step-by-step run though of the procedure, pain, downtime, and cost).

A consultation is successful when the healthcare provider either meets or goes above the patient's expectations. How you do this can vary but it is always worth using different tools to reinforce what you are saying. After all, people have four distinctive learning types [1]:

- *Visual:* Prefer images, charts and graphs when learning
- *Auditory:* Prefer to listen to information when learning
- *Reading/writing:* Prefer to read and write when learning
- *Kinaesthetic:* Prefer to learn through recreating, practicing, and hands-on experience ('tactile learners')

As 50–70% of the population have affinities to more than one style of learning (multimodal leaners), it is important to include tools during the consultation to cater to all four learning types [1]. How you position yourself in the consultation is important. If possible, it is best to have two separate areas. The first one is more formal, using a desk to enter into a conversation with the patient. You can sit behind the desk or next to the patient; this is a personal choice. Make sure the patient is seated comfortably, with both feet touching the floor, to avoid the feeling of being trapped. This is where most of the conversation takes place, including going through the patient questionnaire, initial assessment, and root cause education. This would be ideal for those with an affinity to auditory learning behaviour.

The second area is the treatment couch. Use this area to physically assess the patient and demonstrate how your treatments will work; you can even ask the patient to hold a mirror so that they can then both see and listen to what you are saying. Some healthcare professionals may ask the patient to demonstrate what they would like to achieve (patients will typically pinch certain areas of their face to demonstrate an area that needs volumising or pull their skin to demonstrate an area that needs lifting). If you have demonstration products (e.g. threads or different thickness of dermal fillers), it would be good to let the patient feel the products that you will be using for their procedure. This part of the consultation would be ideal for those with an affinity to visual, auditory, and kinaesthetic learning behaviours.

Before and after pictures demonstrating your work are vital to helping educate your patient, especially for visual and kinaesthetic learners. Make sure you provide context to the picture with information on the model and information on the treatment (for reading learners). Your before and after pictures should be presented in a professional way and it would benefit your business if you could invest time in understanding photography, lighting, and the equipment required to achieve consistently high-quality pictures. Good quality before and after pictures are priceless when it comes to demonstrating your work for consultation and marketing. A review from the model should always accompany the picture (another great tool for reading learners). Some healthcare professionals may prefer to have patient information leaflets for specific treatments that patients can take home to read.

When educating a patient, it is also important to check that they understand and agree with what you are saying. By asking questions that require a 'yes' or 'no' answer, you can gauge whether the patient understands your explanation and if 'yes' is the response, you start to build momentum with the patient. The more times you achieve a 'soft yes', the more likely the patient will agree to the treatment plan you propose a few minutes later. Table 1.1 sets out some common patient concerns and strategies you can use to help your patients overcome them.

TABLE 1.1

Common Patient Concerns and Strategies to Overcome Them

Common Concern	Strategy
Fear of pain during treatment	Testimonial from patients or members of staff who had the same procedure
Fear of complications from treatment	Data on safety of the procedure
Fear of bad results	Before and after photos
Fear of unnatural results	Photos of successful patients
Fear of long downtime	Data on recovery times and aftercare instructions
Fear of needing frequent re-treatments	Data on length of results
Fear of cost	Payment plans or staggered stages of treatment

After presenting treatment options and education, the next steps of the consultation should be evaluating the patient's expectations and treatment options and obtaining the patient's commitment to schedule treatment appointments. These can be done by simply asking the following questions:

- What are your thoughts on the treatment plan?
- What appeals to you about the treatment plan?
- Do you have any further questions for me?
- When would you like to start with the treatments?

How Do I Monitor If My Consultations Are Working?

KPIs measure areas of performance that are critical to either a person or a business performing well. It is important you record your KPIs over time to evaluate performance and progression and to predict future trends.

In order to measure KPIs accurately and obtain meaningful results, a patient questionnaire (with a section for the patient to state the reason for their visit, i.e. apparent want) must be handed out to all new patients prior to consultation with the healthcare professional (see Aesthetic Interest Questionnaire above). At the end of each day, the following data must be recorded onto a spreadsheet:

- Patient's apparent want
- Number of new patients for consultation
- Number of questionnaires handed out
- Number of treatments after consultation (including additional treatments from upselling opportunities from the treatment plan)

Four KPIs that are relevant to the consultation process are as follows:

- *Consultation conversion rate:* This allows you to monitor how many of your patient consultations convert to a paid for treatment. This rate gives you the ability to measure the impact of change within your consultation process, e.g. by adding before and after pictures. This can be measured as a direct percentage of patients who went on to have treatments. For example, if you had ten patients for consultations and eight of them ended up having treatments, your consultation conversion rate is 80%.
- *Upsell conversion rate:* The aim of this calculation is to obtain an average number of treatments you can upsell by creating a personalised treatment plan for your patient per consultation. The upsell conversion rate can be calculated by

$$\frac{\text{Number of treatments identified}}{\text{Number of patients booked for consultation}} \times 100\%$$

Using the above example, if those eight converted patients had multiple treatments (based on your personalised treatment plans) with a total number of procedures of 15, your upsell conversion rate per consultation would be $15 \div 10 \times 100\%$, which would be 150%.

- *Conversion rate per specific treatment:* Relevant to the transactional method of consultation, this allows you to see which treatment interests convert better than others.
- *12-month patient spending.* The better the patient is educated at the start, the greater potential for a higher spending. By recording this over 12 months, you will be able to see if how you educate your patients is meeting your expectations.

The Challenge

Being financially successful is important but seeing a patient's reaction when their results exceed their expectations is very rewarding. Ask yourself this question: what was your best moment in medical aesthetics? Was it when a patient agreed to a £10k treatment plan or was it when a patient couldn't stop smiling because of the results you achieved for them?

If you look after your patients, then the rest of your business will follow. Don't be afraid to try new things and open the horizon because successful businesses are built on reputation, and reputation is formed from honest, personal, and caring consultations.

The challenge is simple. To truly be good at something takes passion, dedication, and willingness to change. How will you apply this to how you consult going forward?

Psychological Assessment in Aesthetics

Aesthetics is very subjective and there is no 'one template fits all' approach when it comes to aesthetics ideal. Sometimes, the decision to have an aesthetics treatment can be a difficult one that is influenced by many external factors. As medical aesthetics procedures are initiated by the patient, it is essential that we recognise the complex psychological milieu behind the decision. During consultation, the patient's general demeanour and personality must be evaluated and the patient's true motive must also be identified. This will help us make the decision whether the patient is suitable for treatment, as many psychological disturbances can be concealed. If this assessment is not carried out thoroughly, we risk selecting patients that are not ideal; even the correct and the best treatment would produce the 'wrong' result.

Anxiety can be common at first meeting and can hamper information retention and expression. Additionally, anxiety can also affect comprehension of goals, benefits, and complications of a treatment. As described above, it is important when educating patients to check that they understand and agree with you. This can be carried out by asking questions that require a 'yes' or 'no' answer.

The prevalence of body dysmorphic disorder (BDD) in aesthetics can be as high as 53% [2]. Hence, appropriate psychological assessment and a system for subsequent referral to mental health professionals (psychologists or psychiatrists) must be in place for each healthcare professional.

Some characteristics of ideal patients for aesthetics procedures include:

- *No obvious psychopathology:* Ideal candidates for medical aesthetics procedures should have good mental health, free from appearance anxiety and BDD.
- *Clearly defined target areas:* Suitable patients will have clear aesthetic goals that they want to achieve and are not in a rush to improve all target areas or skin concerns at once.
- *Realistic expectations:* Patients who are suitable for non-surgical interventions are those who are looking to make minor changes to their appearance. Generally, they opt for a gradual improvement over time rather than drastic changes in a short time frame; they want to look the best version of themselves and not trying to turn back the clock. They also understand that results would vary according to lifestyle and that all procedures carry some risks.

- *Has motivation from or to self:* This is an important point as suitable candidates should not feel pressured, coerced, or bullied into having a procedure. They must not turn to medical aesthetics as a way to solve underlying life issues or during difficult times (e.g. separation or eating disorder). Furthermore, they must not assume that their lives would change if they look better (e.g. relationship, social skills, or job prospect). A suitable patient understands that they have full control of their body and appearance and is clear about why they want to change the way they look. They would only have a procedure because they want to improve their overall well-being and not to please someone else.

Patients with clinical signs of mental disturbances, such as self-mutilation, major depression, and suicidal thoughts, should be avoided and referred for psychological or psychiatric assessment.

There are some in-clinic tools to help healthcare professionals with psychological assessments.

- COPS questionnaire for BDD [3]

   This questionnaire can be used as a screening questionnaire to help diagnose BDD. Note that only a trained healthcare professional can make a diagnosis of BDD, but the questionnaire can help guide you when assessing patients for aesthetics. The questionnaire assumes that the patient does not have a disfigurement or a defect that is easily noticeable. The questionnaire can also be used as a measure of severity of BDD in confirmed cases, to see whether the symptoms have improved or not with treatment. The questionnaire consists of nine questions. The scoring range is 0–72, where 72 is the most severe. A score below 30 is considered unlikely to have BDD.

- Appearance Anxiety Inventory [4]

   The questionnaire has just 10 items and helps score the level of appearance anxiety in patients. The range is 0–40, with a score of 40 being the most severe. A score above 20 is indicative of high risk of clinical problems.

- The STEP approach for psychological assessment [5]

The STEP (Stress, Target, Envision, Proactive) approach is a quick and easy method of assessing the patient's overall motivation during consultation. The four simple steps include:

- *Stress:* The healthcare professional identifies the patient's stressors and their importance (e.g. frown lines). Ensure that you can see those stressors and make sure that they are realistic, not exaggerated. This is a good time to ask if anyone else had told them that they should have the procedure (if this had not already been done).
- *Target:* Allow the patient to describe their aesthetics goals and prioritise specific treatment areas. Ensure that the target is realistic and achievable. It is recommended to focus on one target at a time.
- *Envision:* The healthcare professional asks the patient to envision how their self-perception, emotions, and life would be different or better after a treatment. This is a good time to evaluate whether the patient's answer is realistic or a fantasy. If it is realistic, are you able to deliver the treatment and meet the patient's expectations?
- *Proactive:* If the goals are clear, realistic, and achievable, the healthcare professional should be proactive and devise a specific treatment plan for the patient.

The threshold for psychological referral should be low. If required, the referral should be positioned as an adjunct and becomes a part of the patient's journey to build confidence, to better understand their appearance, and to alleviate any external stress factors (e.g. social media influence).

Conclusion

Balancing patient selection, financial success, and exceeding patient expectations can be a difficult task. A comprehensive and detailed cosmetic consultation can provide you with the right tools to help navigate your way when done correctly. First impression works both ways in medical aesthetics; the initial consultation is your chance to impress a potential patient – but equally, it is also your opportunity to judge whether or not the patient is a suitable candidate for treatment.

REFERENCES

1. Leite WL, Svinicki M, Shi, Y, "Attempted validation of the scores of the VARK: Learning styles inventory with multitrait–multimethod confirmatory factor analysis models," *Educational and Psychological Measurement*, vol. 70, no. 2, pp. 323–339, 2009.
2. Bjornsson AS, Didie ER, Phillips KA, "Body dysmorphic disorder," *Dialogues in Clinical Neuroscience*, vol. 12, no. 2, pp. 221–232, 2010.
3. Veale D, Ellison N, Werner TG, Dodhia R, Serfaty MA, Clarke A, "Development of a cosmetic procedure screening questionnaire (COPS) for body dysmorphic disorder," *Journal of Plastic Reconstructive and Aesthetic Surgery*, vol. 65, no. 4, pp. 530–532, 2012.
4. Veale D, Eshkevari E, Kanakam N, Ellison N, Costa A, Werner T, "The appearance anxiety inventory. Behavioural and cognitive psychotherapy," *Behavioural and Cognitive Psychotherapy*, vol. 42, no. 5, pp. 605–616, 2014.
5. Elsaie ML, "Psychological approach in cosmetic dermatology for optimum patient satisfaction," *Indian Journal of Dermatology*, vol. 55, no. 2, pp. 127–129, 2010.

2

The Skin

**Sue Ann Chan, Sarah Whitehead, Darika de Bacq Rose,
Alexander Parys, and Vincent Wong**

CONTENTS

The skin is the largest organ of the body consisting of three main layers including the epidermis, dermis, and the subcutaneous layer [1, 2]. The epidermis (Figure 2.1) is the outermost layer of the skin composed of mainly keratinocyte cells which forms 80% of the epidermis and other cells including melanocytes (pigment cells), Merkel cells (mechanoreceptors located in sites of high tactile sensitivity), and Langerhans cells (responsible for a variety of T-cell responses for our immune system) [1]. In darker skin-type individuals, the heavier pigment on the skin can be attributed to a greater production of melanosomes dispersed into the keratinocytes from the melanocytes [1].

The dermis beneath the epidermis (Figure 2.2) consists of connective tissue providing elasticity, pliability, and strength to the skin, holding the structure of the skin together. These include appendageal cells such as the apocrine and eccrine sweat glands, sebaceous glands, the vasculature, and nerve

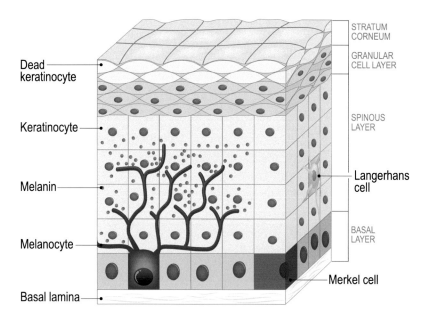

FIGURE 2.1   The epidermis.

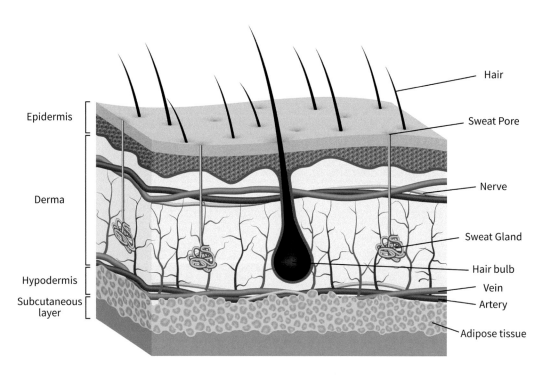

FIGURE 2.2   The epidermis, dermis, and hypodermis.

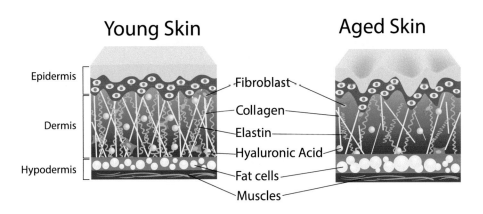

FIGURE 2.3   The structural changes between young and aged skin.

supply to our skin. The principle component of the dermis is collagen, a fibrous protein providing a major stress resistant material to the skin, whilst the elasticity of the skin is provided by protein filaments and elastin [1].

The subcutaneous layer of the skin (also known as hypodermis; see Figure 2.2) lies beneath the dermis and is composed of fat and connective tissue. This layer provides energy and insulation to the skin and also gives contour and shape to our body [2].

Cutaneous ageing can be classified into photo-ageing on the surface of the skin and structural changes affecting the underlying structures and layers of the skin including the subcutaneous tissue which can be regarded as the most substantial influencer to soft-tissue changes/contour of the face and body [3, 4].

Biochemically, photo-ageing causes reduction in the production of elastic fibres and type 1 collagen (which is the predominant type of collagen in the extracellular matrix [ECM] of the human skin) and type 3 collagen in the skin [5]. This mechanism is thought to be induced by metalloproteinase induction induced by ultraviolet (UV) exposure, upregulating transcription factors AP-1 and NF-KB which degrades collagen and elastin in the ECM. The main modality of insult to the skin from the environment is the oxidative stress that is created on the skin by reducing the enzymatic (glutathione peroxidase, glutathione oxidase, superoxide dismutase, catalase) and non-enzymatic (vitamin C, E, glutathione) antioxidant capacity [6]. Fibroblast can also be reduced or damaged by reactive oxidative species (ROS) which has been shown to cause skin ageing in the photo-damaged skin [7].

Clinically, the ageing skin would manifest as thinner epidermis, whilst our dermis becomes less structured and less dense. The loss of fat in the subcutaneous layer also causes our face and body to lose its shape and contour (Figure 2.3).

Collagen, Elastin, and Hyaluronic Acid Production

Collagen is produced from fibroblast in the dermis and is essential for firm, healthy, and youthful looking skin. The dermis consists mainly of Collagen-1 and Collagen-3 fibres to a lesser extent [7]. The collagen fibres can be reduced significantly with increased collagen degradation due to oxidative stress products such as metalloproteinases, serine, and other proteinases due to chronological ageing and photo-ageing. Alongside this, production of collagen by fibroblast also reduces with age [7].

Elastin is a highly elastic protein in connective tissue that allows tissues in our body to resume its shape after stretching. With chronological ageing, the production of elastin is reduced and the degradation

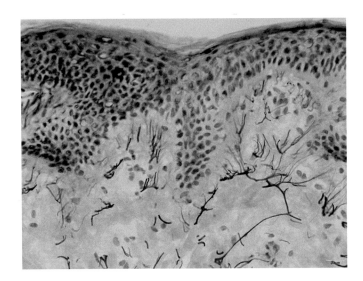

FIGURE 2.4 (×20 magnification) Photo-protected skin of young volunteer: fine elastin fibres in superficial dermis attached to basement membrane with minimal photo-damaged elastin fibres in the dermis. (Courtesy of Faculty of Biology, Medicine and Health, University of Manchester.)

of elastin increases [8]. With UV-induced photo-ageing, a massive accumulation of elastotic material occurs in the upper and mid-dermis, causing solar elastosis of the skin where the tensile strength of the skin is reduced (Figures 2.4 and 2.5).

Hyaluronic acid (HA) is a key molecule in our skin which functions to retain skin hydration with its unique capacity to retain water [9]. HA is synthesised by specific enzymes called HA synthetase usually found in the inner surface of plasma membranes. HA is then extruded through pore-like structures into the extracellular space. The metabolism of HA in our body is extremely complex [9]. With photo-ageing, HA can be degraded via a free-radical non-enzymatic mechanism.

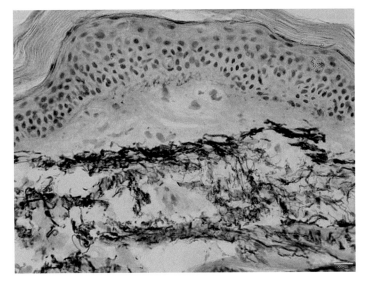

FIGURE 2.5 (×20 magnification) Photo-exposed skin of older volunteer: abundant photo-damaged elastic fibres in dermis. (Courtesy of Faculty of Biology, Medicine and Health, University of Manchester.)

Wound Healing and Rejuvenation

Regeneration and tissue repair occur following tissue injury in our body via a series of molecular and biochemical sequences [10]. These mechanisms form the basis of skin rejuvenation in cosmetic procedures. There are three main stages in wound healing: the inflammatory stage, followed by the proliferative stage, and subsequently the remodelling stage [10].

Inflammatory Stage (~Within the First 48 Hours)

When tissue injury occurs, a vascular response ensues causing aggregation of blood cells including platelets and fibrin deposits in the site of injury. These responses form a clot to seal the area of injury re-establishing homeostasis. This is followed by a series of biochemical and molecular inflammatory response to recruit immunological cells to the area of concern. Monocytes from the infiltrating blood stream differentiate into macrophages which release growth factors including platelet-derived growth factors (PDGFs) and vascular endothelial growth factors (VEGFs). This is an important step in the transition from inflammatory stage to proliferative stage in wound healing.

Proliferative Stage (~48 Hours to 14th Day)

This stage is essential in closure of the wounded site, establishing a viable barrier via angiogenesis, fibroplasia, and re-epithelisation. Following vascular angiogenesis, granulation tissue begins to form from approximately day 4 after the injury forming new stroma. This is followed by fibroplasia characterised by the formation of fibroblast, the main agent responsible for the proliferation of new matrix.

Remodelling Stage (~2–3 Weeks)

The remodelling stage is essential in reorganisation, degradation, and re-synthesis of the extracellular matrix. This stage attempts to recover the normal tissue structure of the skin. The granulation tissue is gradually remodelled, forming a scar tissue that is less vascular, with increased amounts of collagen fibres with resolution of initial inflammation. This occurs via various molecular and biochemical pathway leading to emigration of cells and cell death via apoptosis.

Within the field of aesthetic medicine, the concept of wound healing forms the basis of many skin treatments. By causing controlled and limited damage to the skin, we can effectively stimulate the skin to regenerate and repair itself. This can help with the production of collagen, restoring moisture, eliminating sagginess, maintaining skin thickness and elasticity, and reducing inflammation and other skin imperfections such as pigmentation. Such treatments can be divided into three main categories:

- Topical and surface treatments
- Energy-based treatments
- Mesotherapy treatments

Topical and Surface Treatments

Topical and surface treatments are easy to perform and can have a visible impact on the skin. These treatments are often the 'starting point' for patients considering treatments to improve their facial appearance, especially younger patients who want to prevent the signs of ageing (prejuvenation). Within this chapter, topical and surface treatments will include:

- Vitamin C
- Retinol

- Skin peels
- Dermaplaning
- Microdermabrasion

Vitamin C

Vitamin C, which also goes by the names ascorbic acid and L-ascorbic acid, is one of the best anti-ageing ingredients to use on the skin. Not only does vitamin C promote collagen synthesis, it is also a potent antioxidant that protects the skin from free radicals caused by sun exposure.

What Does It Do?

Vitamin C evens out skin tone, brightens a dull complexion, fades age spots, and boosts the production of collagen, improves rough texture, fine lines, acne scars, and general dullness. It neutralises free radicals, aids your skin's natural regeneration process, which helps your body repair damaged skin cells. Studies have shown that vitamin C effectiveness increases when combined with other antioxidants, such as vitamin E. Together they can double the protection against UV and free-radical damage [11].

How Does It Work?

Vitamin C is a key component for skin-brightening, as it inhibits melanin production and brown spots by evening out skin tone. It keeps inflammation at bay, and furthermore, it may even help protect the skin from pre-cancerous changes from UV light exposure by neutralising free radicals [12]. Vitamin C is highly acidic and very bitter, so when applied to the skin, the skin is triggered to 'heal' itself by accelerating the production of collagen and elastin [13].

Who Is a Suitable Candidate?

Vitamin C has an excellent safety profile and most people can use topical vitamin C for an extended period of time without experiencing any adverse reactions [14].

What Are the Benefits?

- Safe for most skin types
- Hydrating
- Brightening
- Reduces redness and even out your skin tone
- Fades hyperpigmentation
- Reduces the appearance of under-eye circles

What Are the Limitations?

If you have sensitive skin or suffer from allergies, it is recommended that you start with a lower concentration or test an area first to make sure that no allergy exists.

Pearls of Wisdom

Vitamin C is notoriously prone to oxidising, meaning that it can break down when it is exposed to light or air.

Retinol

Since its discovery and entrance into the skincare scene in 1971, this humble ingredient has quickly taken on a reputation as a cure-all for every possible skincare concern. Retinol, better known as Vitamin A, helps to smooth out imperfections and reduce the appearance of lines and wrinkles. It can also help to reduce the appearance of age spots, pigmentation, and sun-damage.

What Does It Do?

Retinol is considered to be the gold-standard ingredient in skincare because it alters the behaviour of aged cells, so they act in a more youthful manner. Retinol activates your skin cells by stimulating the production of new blood vessels and speeding up skin cell renewal, acting as an anti-ageing superhero. It helps to improve the look of fine lines, sun damage, and wrinkles. As a result, the skin looks fuller, firmer, and more radiant, with fewer visible lines.

How Does It Work?

When retinol converts into retinoic acid, it induces exfoliation which allows skin cells to function normally and continue regular cell renewal. Retinol is an antioxidant, which means it helps to neutralise substances called free radicals that destroy healthy skin cells. By neutralising free radicals, retinol calms the skin, decreasing stress factors that may damage the skin [15].

Who Is a Suitable Candidate?

Retinol, or vitamin A, is best for 30+ skin with fine lines and wrinkles; however, you can start using retinols younger if you want to, although younger skin types may not see the effects as much as older skin types as they have fewer age concerns. Retinol can enhance collagen production to prevent the formation of future lines and wrinkles [16].

What Are the Benefits?

- Prevent wrinkles due to its minimising effect, as well as smooth out existing fine lines and wrinkles
- Brighten dull skin by exfoliating at a cellular level, which results in brighter and smoother new skin
- Regulate oily skin and minimise breakouts
- Fade dark age spots, sunspots, and hyperpigmentation and even out complexion over time

What Are the Limitations?

If incorporated into a skincare regimen too quickly or used too often, flakiness, dryness, and even some breakouts can occur. Typically, it takes a little time for the skin to adjust. It is recommended to avoid retinol during pregnancy and while breastfeeding because it has the potential to cause birth defects, although the risk is low.

Pearls of Wisdom

Encapsulated retinol causes less irritation due to slow release mechanism.

Skin Peels

Chemical peels, also known as chemoexfoliation or derma-peeling, involve the application of a chemical solution that is used to rejuvenate the skin. Recipes for peelings date back to medical texts of old Egypt.

The oldest medical papyri contain recipes for 'improving beauty of the skin' and 'removing wrinkles' by use of agents such as salt and soda. The Egyptian Queen Cleopatra (69–30 BC) is said to have taken baths in donkey's milk to improve the beauty of her skin [17].

What Does It Do?

Chemical peels are used to correct skin irregularities in texture, such as fine lines, and colour, such as spots caused by sun damage. Peels vary in strength and are characterised by the different kinds of acids used. Superficial peels remove the outer layer of the epidermis, medium depth peels work deeper in the epidermal layer, and deep peels extend deep into the lower dermis layer of the skin. As the skin goes through a healing process, new cells are made, and there is a greater collagen production which helps to achieve a more rejuvenated and youthful look.

How Does It Work?

A superficial peel is like a mild 'sandpapering' of the skin and dissolves the dead/flaky skin that clogs up the pores, resulting in a healthier looking complexion. There are several forms of hydroxy acids that are used in superficial peels, but these are the most common:

- *Glycolic acid* is typically derived from sugar cane, it belongs to the alpha hydroxy acid (AHA) family – along with malic, tartaric, and lactic acids. Chemically, it is a small molecule, which means when you put it on the skin, it can penetrate readily [18].
- *Salicylic acid* is a beta hydroxy acid. It is unique amongst the hydroxy acids as it is lipophilic in nature. It is able to penetrate deeper into the oil glands to reduce oil production, clear out pores, and prevent outbreaks. It's a true 'superhero' for acne-prone skin.

The main function of these acids is to exfoliate the pores, ungluing dead cells from each other, creating fresh new skin cells.

The most common acid used in medium depth peels is trichloroacetic acid (TCA).

TCA is a carboxylic acid and a relative to vinegar. It has been around for use in peels for about 20 years and penetrates deeper than the hydroxy acids [19]. When TCA is applied to the skin, it causes protein to precipitate and denature, resulting in keratoagulation (also known as frosting). Once frosting has occurred, the acid needs to be neutralised. When the old skin is peeled off, it exposes a new layer of undamaged skin, which has a smoother texture and more even colour.

Deep peels are generally performed using phenol. Phenol is the strongest of all chemical peels and produces a dramatic result, but a local anaesthetic is required. Continuous heart monitoring is also required as phenol has the potential to cause irregular heartbeats in some patients.

Who Is a Suitable Candidate?

Suitable for all skin types in both men and women. The best candidates are often those with fair, thin skin that has a tendency of fine wrinkling or scarring on the face.

What Are the Benefits?

- Significant improvement in the appearance of fine lines and wrinkles
- Improves acne-prone skin
- Reduces hyperpigmentation caused by sun damage
- Decreases pore size
- Refines texture and tone of the skin
- Reduces the effects of rosacea and acne scarring

What Are the Limitations?

Some deeper peels require significant downtime and are unsuitable for highly pigmented skin, such as those with Asian, Black, and Mediterranean complexions, as they can cause post-inflammatory hyperpigmentation.

Pearls of Wisdom

People who have been known to develop brown discoloration after injury, such as a mild burn, should have a test area peeled first before undergoing a full-face chemical peel.

Dermaplaning

Dermaplaning, also known as microplaning or blading, is a form of mechanical exfoliation, where dead/dry skin cells and the fine vellus hairs on the face (known as peach fuzz) are skimmed away from the outermost layers of the epidermis using a sterile surgical scalpel.

What Does It Do?

Dermaplaning brightens the complexion, reduces congestion, reveals radiant glowing skin, and creates pathways for the absorption of skin peels and products to be more effective.

How Does It Work?

A sterile medical blade is used to glide across the skin in an upwards direction. This is done carefully and progressively until the whole face has been treated. Dermaplaning triggers the cell regeneration process, which helps to improve, soften, and smooth the appearance of acne scarring, hyper-pigmentation, and sun damage. Absorption of peels and serums is much more effective on the newly exfoliated skin, resulting in a glowing hair-free appearance.

Who Is a Suitable Candidate?

Anyone who has unwanted facial hair and anyone who wants exfoliation will benefit. Dermaplaning is also great for anyone who is unable to use certain products or other exfoliating treatments, such as pregnant women or those with super-sensitive skin. It is an alternative way to lightly resurface the skin and is safe for all skin types.

What Are the Benefits?

- Provides deeper product penetration
- Removes soft facial hair that traps dirt and oils
- Promotes smoother skin
- Safe procedure for removing dead skin cells and 'peach fuzz'
- Reduces the appearance of acne scars
- Diminishes the look of fine lines
- Works on all skin types

What Are the Limitations?

Dermaplaning is a safe, low-risk procedure for most skin types. Side effects are minimal; however, those with sensitive skins may experience slight redness for a few hours of post-treatment. It is not recommended for highly reactive skin, open wounds or raised lesions, or those with rosacea or keratosis pilaris. It should also not be used on inflamed acne as sliding a sharp scalpel over spots can irritate them and worsen existing breakouts.

Pearls of Wisdom

It is important to advise patients to protect their skin with a physical sunblock after the procedure.

Microdermabrasion

Microdermabrasion goes as far back as far as the Ancient Egyptians, who would use sandpaper to soften the appearance of scars. It wasn't until 1985 when the modern machine was developed by Drs Mattioli and Brutto [20].

Microdermabrasion, which is also known as microderm or dermabrasion, is a non-invasive procedure and works by using one of two methods, either gliding a crystal/diamond tipped wand across the skin or by firing highly pressurised crystals across the skin surface, which gently exfoliates the top layer of the epidermis, while simultaneously using suction to draw out dead skin cells and impurities, almost like a human skin vacuum cleaner, leaving the skin cleaner and brighter.

What Does It Do?

Buffing away the dead skin cells leaves the skin looking more radiant and feeling smoother. It can help improve surface texture and very superficial fine lines and wrinkles. The exfoliating technique has an ability to trigger increased levels of collagen and elastin, leading to a fresher appearance and general improvement in the texture of the skin.

How Does It Work?

Movement of these crystals on the skin under pressure loosens and partially removes the outermost epidermal layer of the skin and has a kind of 'sandpapering' effect. When you remove the stratum corneum, the body interprets it as an injury and quickly replaces the lost skin cells with new, healthy ones. The procedure stimulates blood flow, which increases the nutrition delivered to skin cells. This in turn improves cell production, which improves the skin's elasticity and texture.

Who Is a Suitable Candidate?

Microdermabrasion is suitable for all Fitzpatrick skin types and will not cause scarring or colour changes. Fine lines and wrinkles can benefit greatly from microdermabrasion, particularly due to the natural promotion of collagen production. It is a less aggressive procedure compared to traditional dermabrasion and has a quicker recovery time, but can still achieve great results.

What Are the Benefits?

- Improved circulation
- Brighter skin complexion
- Improvement of fine lines and wrinkles
- Reduction of congested pores

What Are the Limitations?

It is not a recommended treatment if you have skin conditions such as rosacea, eczema, active sunburn, herpes, lupus, open sores, psoriasis, fragile capillaries, or widespread acne. This can irritate the skin and cause further breakouts.

Pearls of Wisdom

The absorption rate of topical active ingredients is higher after microdermabrasion.

Energy-Based Treatments

In recent years, energy-based treatments have grown in popularity due to the dramatic changes that they can bring about when it comes to skin quality and skin health. These treatments target the skin beyond the surface and can be useful for a variety of indications, from treating skin diseases to the removal of skin lesions.

Plasma Therapy ('Cold Plasma')

In aesthetics, this treatment can be used for a variety of indications such as improving acne [21], the appearance of scarring, and stretch marks. It may successfully remove cosmetically unacceptable benign skin lesions such as xanthelasmata, seborrhoeic keratosis, and warts [22, 23]. For many aesthetic practitioners, perhaps the most valuable and interesting application is for skin tightening; in face and body but especially in non-surgical blepharoplasty.

How Does It Work?

Delivery of plasma energy onto the skin tissue surface is generated by a tiny electrical arc created from the tip of the device and ionisation of gas in the air [24]. This leads to an instant contraction of the skin tissue at the site of application and also triggers a process termed 'sublimation'. This is where solid turns directly into a gas, without transitioning through a liquid, thus limiting any thermal damage to the treated tissue (compared with other treatments such as radiofrequency [RF] and laser) and enabling tissue removal without excision. Neocollagenesis (the remodelling of fibrillar collagen type III) via fibroblast activation and migration from deep to more superficial dermis alongside cytokine release leads to a regeneration of tissue, represented clinically by skin with decreased laxity and a refreshed cosmetic appearance [25, 26].

Technique

This depends on the device used and treatment indication, but often the skin is prepared with a skin disinfectant and application of a topical anaesthetic cream. Plasma energy may be applied either by discrete spots or continuous spraying (plasma 'shower'). When treating delicate eyelid skin, it is imperative to leave some untreated skin between the treated spots to allow for good wound healing and contraction of the area.

Immediately after treatment there will be contraction of the tissue (not always reflective of the end outcome) and the appearance of brown spots of carbonised tissue to treatment zones which resolve and flake from the skin within 5–7 days [28].

Who Is a Suitable Candidate?

Individuals (without contraindication to treatment) with:

- Excess skin on their upper and lower eyelids [27]
- Photo-damaged skin, fine lines, and skin laxity to face, neck, or body areas
- Stretch marks and scars (not hypertrophic or keloid)
- Acne
- Benign skin lesions

What Are the Benefits?

- No need for general anaesthetic and associated risks
- More affordable to patients than surgical blepharoplasty
- No surgical sutures or scar

- Minimal risk of damage to underlying obicularis musculature
- Relatively low downtime
- Quick, easily tolerable, office-based procedure
- Extremely low running costs once device is purchased and therefore potential for yielding high profit margin per treatment session

What Are the Limitations?

There are several potential contraindications to plasma treatment, some of which may be at the discretion of the medical practitioner depending on their experience and level of skill:

- Pregnancy and breastfeeding, metal implants, pacemakers, treatment with Isotretinoin (Roaccutane), concurrent illness or infection, any skin lesions or breaches in integrity to treatment area, autoimmune conditions, diabetes mellitus, hepatitis, bone disease, epilepsy, cancers, keloid scars.
- Patients with skin Fitzpatrick types 3 and above may be more prone to hyperpigmentation and may not be suitable for this treatment modality, either without skin preparation or at all [24].
- Patient selection is important with non-surgical blepharoplasty as those with significant upper lid subcutaneous fat and hooding may be dissatisfied with aesthetic outcome vs surgery [28].
- Several treatments are often required (sometimes 3+), performed approximately every 6 weeks, to achieve desired results deemed comparable to surgery.
- Complications may include bruising, persistent oedema, infection, persistent erythema, and pigmentation issues. Suboptimal or asymmetric cosmesis is a possible concern and thorough and comprehensive training is key to ensure correct patient selection and usage of the device [28].

Pearls of Wisdom

Direct current plasma devices allow for better depth control and are less likely to cause serious complications (e.g. scarring) compared to alternating current devices.

Laser and Intense Pulsed Light (IPL)

In aesthetic medicine, these devices are used to remove/lessen unwanted hair, treat acne and alleviate acne scarring, remove benign pigmented lesions, unwanted tattoos, erase vascular lesions, thread veins and varicose veins [29]. They can affect rejuvenation by enhancing skin texture and tone, addressing rhytides and tightening skin laxity.

How Does It Work?

The concept of using LASER (Light Amplification by Stimulated Emission of Radiation) to treat skin disorders dates back to the early 1980s [30] when it was noted that light at a particular wavelength could be applied to target a specific area of skin to create an effect, whilst sparing the surrounding tissue. Chromophores within the skin absorb light energy which, once converted into thermal energy, damages the absorptive chromophore thus breaking down the target. The main chromophores which laser and IPL energy can target are haemoglobin, melanin, and water, and it is their effect on each of these which translates into the resulting target outcomes. In simple terms, haemoglobin is targeted for vascular conditions, melanin for pigment conditions, and water for resurfacing, lines, and wrinkles.

There are several broad categories of laser and light therapy [31]:

1. IPL therapy uses a flash lamp light source to emit non-coherent light with wavelengths 515–1200 nm with filters set to allow for the targeting of selective chromophores for melanin vs haemoglobin [32]. Its use of a spectrum of wavelengths allows for penetration to different depths in

the skin to target both dermal and epidermal zones simultaneously. The size of the IPL head is larger than most laser spot sizes, which also allows for more rapid treatment of larger areas. IPL is quite a versatile device which can target many different sizes of blood vessels, pigmented lesions, and hair follicles. This can be therefore be utilised for hair removal, melasma, benign pigmented lesions, thread veins, erythema, and acne and to generate collagen stimulation for aesthetic skin rejuvenation [33].

2. Q-switched lasers use very short pulses of high-intensity laser beams at various wavelengths, e.g. Ruby (694 nm), Alexandrite (755 nm), and ND:YAG (532 or 1064 nm) [34]. These are useful for tattoo removal, birthmarks, benign pigmented lesions such as lentigenes as they are highly pigment selective. Newer variances using a low fluence or subthermolytic Q-switched treatment are increasing in popularity (aiming to disrupt pigment whilst sparing the actual melanocytes and keratinocytes) as they are able to be used with less adverse effect on cosmesis with a higher Fitzpatrick skin type [35]. These lasers are also effective for face and body hair removal.

3. Non-ablative fractionated resurfacing lasers create selective columns of microthermal damage, where treated and untreated areas are mixed in a grid pattern, resulting in less 'downtime' and lower inflammation. These devices target the water chromophore, but create columns of dermal damage whilst maintaining an intact stratum corneum. Neocollagenesis and remodelling are thereby stimulated and this modality is used for aesthetic skin rejuvenation [36].

4. Ablative fractionated resurfacing lasers such as CO_2 and Erbium:YAG lasers cause ablation/removal of the epidermis whilst targeting the dermis to affect neocollagenesis. As the epidermis heals and regrows, the treated area appears smoother and tighter with a fresh 'new' epidermal layer. This is useful for treating scarred skin and for more aggressive photorejuvenation [33].

5. Picosecond lasers are a relatively new design, generating picosecond domain pulses which lead to pigment fragmentation resultant from photoacoustic effects (vs photo thermal), which, in practice, is beneficial for the removal of a wider range of coloured pigment in multicoloured tattoos [37]. It may also be used to treat acne scarring and for skin revitalisation to improve tone, texture, rhytides, and pigmented lesions.

6. Pulsed dye lasers (585 nm) target haemoglobin chromophores and can be used to effectively treat vascular lesions such as haemangiomas, port wine stains, birthmarks, vascular ectasia, and telangiectasia [38].

Technique

For a non-ablative laser or IPL treatment, the skin may be prepared with a topical anaesthetic, and goggles will be worn to protect both the patient's and practitioner's eyes.

The handpiece of the device is placed against the skin surface, and activating the laser or IPL may feel like the snapping of a rubber band against the skin.

Skin surface cooling is applied during treatment and often cool packs immediately post-treatment to soothe and further cool the area.

For ablative laser treatment, the patient may require local anaesthetic injections and intravenous sedation to be able to tolerate the procedure. Skin will need to be protected with a thick balm and even occlusive dressings until the epidermis renews.

Patients must vigilantly protect their treated skin from sun exposure to reduce the risk of post-inflammatory hyperpigmentation.

Who Is a Suitable Candidate?

- Patients looking to treat pigmentation such as solar lentigenes, cosmetically unacceptable benign pigmented lesions, acne scarring, fine lines and rhytides, mild to moderate skin laxity, and uneven skin tone
- Patients desiring tattoo removal or hair removal

- Patients with cosmetically unacceptable vascular lesions such as telangiectasia, birthmarks, and haemangiomas
- Patients with a lighter skin tone (Fitzpatrick I, II, and III), as they will have reduced risk of post-treatment hyperpigmentation
- Patients who will reliably protect their skin from sun exposure following treatment

What Are the Benefits?

- No surgical incisions or scars
- No general anaesthetic
- Minimal downtime from IPL and non-ablative laser treatments
- Some treatments can yield combination results to reduce vascular lesions, pigmented lesions, and skin rhytides and to promote skin rejuvenation simultaneously
- Can be performed on facial skin and body skin and specialised treatments include vulval rejuvenation and vaginal tightening

What Are the Limitations?

Contraindications to treatment would include:

- Pregnancy
- Epilepsy
- Treatment with Isotretinoin within 12 months
- Autoimmune conditions
- Hypertrophic or keloid scarring
- History of cold sores/herpes virus
- Darker skin tones, Fitzpatrick 3, and above need to be treated with caution and dependent on level of expertise of the practitioner and often following preparation of the skin with anti-tyrosinase topical therapy [34]
- For hair removal, laser and IPL are ineffective with white, red, grey, and blonde hairs [33]
- Non-ablative laser resurfacing can precipitate infection (e.g. herpes simplex flare) and post-inflammatory hyperpigmentation
- Mild erythema and oedema are relatively common, but this usually resolves within hours or days

Ablative lasers have the most potential for significant adverse effects [38]:

- Treated skin may be erythematous, itchy, and oedematous, and this erythema may persist for some time following ablative laser treatment
- Infection post-treatment with bacteria, fungus, or virus, particularly herpes simplex, can be a problem. Acne may be an issue following ablative laser due to occlusive topicals and dressing usage
- Post-treatment hypopigmentation or post-inflammatory hyperpigmentation
- There is a minor risk of permanent scarring and ectropion when treatment is performed near the lower eyelid

Pearls of Wisdom

Laser technology is a rapidly evolving industry and innovative research into other benefits, e.g. the potential to use laser as a drug delivery system (e.g. hydroquinone for melasma and PIH, platelet-rich plasma [PRP] for rejuvenation) is currently ongoing [39].

LED Therapy (Light-Emitting Diode Therapy, a Type of Low-Level Light Therapy [LLLT])

In aesthetic medicine, light emitting diodes (LEDs) can be used to improve the appearance of photo-aged skin by photobiomodulation, a non-thermal (vs radio frequency and focused ultrasound, which create a thermal injury) and non-ablative mechanism. Depending on the type of light used, this process stimulates collagen synthesis, fibroblast proliferation, growth factors, and the extra cellular matrix via 'charging' the cellular mitochondria. This translates to improved skin texture (appearing more hydrated, smoother, brighter), lifting, tightening, and reduction of rhytides and skin laxity. Redness and inflammatory acne vulgaris lesions may also be improved.

How Does It Work?

Phototherapy uses non-invasive, non-UV (ultraviolet), and non-thermal light to achieve a desired therapeutic outcome. The clinical evidence for this modality (originally developed decades ago by NASA for its potential to assist in plant photosynthesis and then wound healing) has grown in the past few years to strongly support the use of LEDs at particular wavelengths of light: blue (415 nm), red (633 nm), and near-infrared (830 nm) in dermatological and aesthetic practice.

Blue light is useful in the management of acne vulgaris by harnessing a process of activating porphyrins which are endogenous within the skin, leading to free-radical formation which then destroys the gram negative *Propionibacterium acnes* implicated in this condition, without usage of topical or oral antibiotics. Blue light also appears to help regulate sebaceous glands/sebum production and improve skin clarity.

Red light is the regenerative wavelength in the spectrum, increasing cellular ATP (energy) to boost faster regeneration. It is absorbed by the fibroblasts in the skin to accelerate collagen and elastin synthesis and also enhances blood flow to increase oxygen availability and lymphatic flow to eliminate toxins. A treatment under a medical grade device with red light may give patients an instant 'glow' and radiance to the skin, alongside a feeling of well-being.

Near infrared light is a deeply penetrating wavelength shown to speed up wound healing, creating a significantly higher and better aligned collagen and elastin fibre density, a thicker and more cellular epidermal layer and a better organised stratum corneum than untreated skin. It triggers anti-inflammatory processes to reduce redness and reduce skin irritation and also helps the appearance of hyperpigmentation.

Red and near infrared lights work best when used synergistically, and some devices (e.g. Dermalux Triwave, Dermalux Flex MD) are able to combine a blue light treatment with the other two wavelengths.

Technique

One of the great advantages of LED therapy is that the treatment is not time consuming for the practitioner. Once the patient has been made comfortable under the device and parameters for treatment set, they may be left to relax and enjoy the therapy for 20–30 minutes. It is a pain free and pleasant sensation, and patients often enter a state of deep relaxation or sleep, an additional restorative benefit.

Who Is a Suitable Candidate?

- Any patient wishing for aesthetic rejuvenation of skin
- Acne vulgaris (not concurrently using photosensitising agent, e.g. Roaccutane)
- Wound healing (or post-iatrogenic injury such as ablative laser or microneedling)
- Rosacea/redness
- Pigmentation
- After other rejuvenation procedures to decrease 'downtime' (erythema, oedema) and potentially optimise results

What Are the Benefits?

- Few contraindications and side effects
- Non-invasive
- Painless, pleasant treatment
- Relatively low cost to patient and minimal usage of physician's time
- Can be used as a standalone or as an adjunct to other aesthetic procedures

What Are the Limitations?

Several treatments are usually required to obtain significant results when used as a stand-alone treatment. Protocols may advise twice weekly sessions of 20 or 30 minutes (device dependent) up to 10 weeks' duration.

Pearls of Wisdom

Photodynamic therapy (PDT) has been used for many years in dermatology to treat various conditions related to photodamage such as superficial basal cell carcinoma and Bowen's Disease (squamous cell carcinoma in situ); this treatment modality also has a potential place in aesthetic medicine to rejuvenate photoaged skin, improving appearance in texture and tone. GlycoAla is a novel new photodynamic (light activated) gel for aesthetic use with red light to decrease pore size, improve clarity and sebum control, and reduce the appearance of fine lines and photodamage.

High-Intensity Focused Ultrasound (HIFU)

In aesthetics, this technology is used for non-invasive skin lifting and tightening, and also for non-invasive fat reduction for the submental area or body contouring. The concept of HIFU is well established in various medical specialties for many years, being used for treating tumours, kidney stones, and uterine fibroids, but first described for use in aesthetic medicine in 2007, for its potential in non-invasive facial rejuvenation and body contouring [40], and the technology was approved by the United States Food and Drug Administration in 2009 for use in brow lifting, and to improve lines and wrinkles in the décolletage area in 2014. Other uses are considered 'off-label'.

How Does It Work?

The principle of HIFU treatment is to selectively induce cellular damage and volume reduction of the targeted area by means of coagulation. The high-intensity ultrasound energy generates microthermal lesions at the specific tissue site, which causes microcoagulation zones from the deep dermis to the superficial musculoaponeurotic system (SMAS) to affect a gradual tightening of the skin through collagen contraction and remodelling [41].

For body contouring, the energy targets adipose tissue to affect thermal coagulation, necrosis, and cell death within the adipocytes. The contents of these ruptured adipocytes (mainly triglycerides) are dispersed into the interstitial tissues before being transported by the lymphatic system. The actual adipocyte cells are resorbed 8–18 weeks after treatment [42].

Techniques

Topical anaesthetic cream may be applied to the treatment area and in some cases, pretreatment medication to control pain. Then, after cleansing, an ultrasound gel will be applied before the device is placed against the skin. The device will be adjusted to target the correct area and depth for treatment, and ultrasound energy will be delivered in pulses for usually between 30 and 90 minutes, dependent on treatment.

Most patients will experience only mild, temporary side effects, such as discomfort, oedema, ecchymosis, erythema, and paraesthesia resolving within 1–2 weeks [43].

Who Is a Suitable Candidate?

- Patients with mild to moderate skin laxity and mild lipoptosis. Younger patients typically yield more significant results [41]
- For body contouring, patients wanting to treat adiposity in particular areas such as abdomen, thighs, and hips
- Patients with skin laxity
- Patients wishing for combination of both fat reduction and skin tightening [44]

What Are the Benefits?

- No general anaesthetic or surgical scars
- Relatively low downtime, any side effects mentioned above usually fully resolve within 1–2 weeks [43]
- High level of patient satisfaction with correct patient selection [45]

What Are the Limitations?

Contraindications to treatment include:

- Pregnancy or breastfeeding
- Heart conditions/pacemaker
- Anticoagulant medication
- Cancer or history of cancer within 5 years
- Metal implants to area of treatment
- Diabetes
- Epilepsy
- Autoimmune conditions
- Transplant
- Liver or kidney impairment
- Systemic Isotretinoin within 6 months

The treatment area must not have been subjected to thread lifts within 6 months or Botulinum toxin or HA fillers within 2 weeks of HIFU procedure.

Pearls of Wisdom

For body contouring, weight should be stable with BMI below 30. HIFU should not be used as an alternative to healthy diet or weight loss [44].

For facial treatment, patients with BMI above 30, extensive skin ptosis/laxity, heavy lipoptosis with jowling and those with marked platsymal banding tend to have less satisfactory outcomes and may be best served with surgical intervention [41].

Radiofrequency

RF devices can be used to address areas of skin laxity and wrinkles, in a non- or minimally invasive way. This includes treatment of periorbital rhytids, lower cheek jowl, nasolabial folds, marionette lines, brow lifting, lower lid tightening, scarring, cheek laxity, neck rejuvenation, and body skin laxity. Also, this modality can be used to treat active acne as well as acne scarring [46] and axillary hyperhidrosis.

How Does It Work?

RF is an alternating electrical current applied to create an electromagnetic field. It includes any electromagnetic frequency within the range of 3 kHz to 300 MHz [47]. It can be monopolar (using a single probe placed on the skin, although this modality is no longer used in newer devices), bipolar (two electrodes applied to the treatment area), or multipolar [48].

Depth of penetration of the RF energy can be controlled to target specific tissue depths (such as papillary dermis, reticular dermis, and fascia superficialis) [49], and delivery may also be varied by device platform to provide fractional (sublative) energy (where a microneedle handpiece is used to physically ablate the skin and deliver a deeper bipolar RF), phase controlled RF or even combination RF, where additional techniques such as infrared light, vacuum, massage, LED, HIFU, and micro-focused ultrasound are incorporated to increase the effects of tightening and skin rejuvenation [50].

The aim of the treatment is to heat the dermis to a point where therapeutics effect occurs but without damage to the surrounding tissues. Ablative RF combines the deep tissue stimulation and neocollagenesis with the additional benefit of ablative epidermal resurfacing.

Technique

The aim with RF is to heat the target (usually dermis or sometimes subcutaneous tissue) whilst protecting the epidermis by keeping it 39–42°C. Some devices use a single touch, whereas others require the treatment head or probe to be circulated or swept over the area.

Devices and thus protocols vary, but often a fine layer of ultrasound gel may be applied to the epidermis to improve the contact between skin and handpiece. A treatment area is mapped out to ensure no 'cold spots'/untreated areas occur during preheating and therapeutic treatment time, and technique is consistent to also avoid 'hotspots'/overtreated areas.

Minimally invasive treatment may require sedation and tumescent local anaesthesia, but non-invasive RF is usually well tolerated by patients.

Who Is a Suitable Candidate?

Ideally, patients have mild/moderate skin laxity and mild rhytides, and are between the ages of 35 and 60 [50].

There are several indications, and these are expanding with the ever-increasing portfolio of available devices to include:

- Facial, neck, and body skin laxity and rhytides
- Brow lifting
- Scar reduction (atrophic, acne)
- Acne
- Axillary hyperhidrosis
- Vulval rejuvenation [51]

What Are the Benefits?

- No general anaesthetic or surgical scarring
- Can be used on patients with previous surgery, fillers, and neurotoxin treatment
- Can be used on patients with beards/facial hair without concern of subsequent hair loss
- Minimal downtime with non-invasive RF treatment, usually erythema and mild oedema resolving over hours

What Are the Limitations?

Contraindications to treatment with RF include:

- Pregnancy
- Electronic or metal containing implants (e.g. pacemaker, hip prosthesis)
- Malignancy (active or recent)
- Immunosuppressive agents

Relative contraindications include:

- Diabetes mellitus
- Systemic retinoid (e.g. Roaccutane) within 6 months
- Topical retinoid use (discontinue 2 weeks prior to treatment)
- Topical corticosteroids (discontinue at least 8 weeks prior to RF treatment)
- Systemic Steroid use (within 12 months)
- Excessive skin laxity/photodamage

Complications of treatment may be minimal with cautious treatment in the hands of an experienced physician. Thermal injury and burns may occur if excess energy is used or contact with a specific area is prolonged.

Pearls of Wisdom

Modern devices will have built in temperature sensors to prevent thermal injuries and burns, but with some older monopolar devices, unintentional treatment of subcutaneous fat in the face can lead to lipodystrophy/atrophy and cosmetically unacceptable depressions [52].

Mesotherapy Treatments

The phrase 'beauty is skin deep', according to the Cambridge Dictionary [53], is used to say that a person's character is more important than how they look. However, in aesthetics, the phrase can perhaps be interpreted in a more literal sense; many patients focus on lines and wrinkles from volume loss but fail to address the largest organ of the body – the skin itself. Studies have demonstrated that skin texture, pigmentation, and elasticity affect the perception of facial age, health, and attractiveness [54, 55]. Therefore, if we truly wish to rejuvenate a person's external appearance, we must also focus on optimising skin texture.

With ageing, there is a reduction in dermal fibroblast activity, and as a result, a reduction in production of HA, collagen, and other components of the extracellular matrix [56], leading to less youthful looking skin (see Figure 2.3).

How Does It Work?

Mesotherapy is a method of introducing microdroplets of products into the superficial layers of the skin and therefore allows active and essential ingredients to come directly into contact with the dermal fibroblast cells, with the aim of enhancing skin quality by improving or maintaining fibroblast function, boosting extracellular matrix component biosynthesis [57]. These mesotherapy products can contain ingredients ranging from HA, vitamins, minerals, and amino acids, to growth factors and PRP. The method of delivering these into the skin can also vary – such as microdroplet boluses with needles, microneedling with a handheld device, plasma shower, or even the 'no needle' injector.

Techniques

- *Nappage technique:* The practitioner manually injects a series of micro-injections into the superficial dermal layer (usually 1–2 mm deep) using a fine gauge needle, creating tiny papules of product at each point.

- *Microneedling pen device* (e.g. SkinPen, DermaPen): These electronic devices use a disposable cartridge which contains multiple ultra-fine sterile needles and then use a motor to insert these into the skin. Product is not directly dispensed through these needles, they instead create micro-channels in the skin which allow the product to be absorbed. The depth of penetration is usually adjustable between 0.25 and 2.5 mm to allow for variability in skin thickness, or for deeper penetration if targeting scarring. In addition, these micro-injuries caused by the microneedling stimulate the body's natural wound healing process, which in turn stimulates collagen to improve skin quality [58].

- *Mesotherapy 'gun'* (e.g. Mesogun U225): These devices live up to their name and resemble a mechanised 'gun' with a tip of fine needles which are automatically powered to deliver a series of micro-injections to adjustable depths of the skin. As a hollow needle is used with the option of connecting a syringe of product, this technique can therefore simultaneously infuse the dermis at a much faster rate, with greater accuracy over depth and quantity of dispensed product vs manual injections.

- *Derma-rollers/derma-stamps:* These are devices that contain numerous fine needles on either a cylindrical 'roller' or a stamper. These come in a variety of different depths but are not adjustable as their penetration depth is fixed. These devices are either manually rolled or stamped over the patient's face to create microchannels for the product to penetrate into the skin. One thing to be aware of with derma-rollers is that, due to the cylindrical roller, the needles enter the skin at 45 degrees and exit at a different angle, creating more of a skin 'tear' than a vertical channel, and as a result the collagen that is formed is the more fibrous type II collagen.

- *Handheld needle delivery systems* (e.g. Aquagold, Wow Fusion): These are small disposable devices which have a reservoir that can be filled with product at one end, and a series of ultra-fine needles at the other which are set to a fixed depth of penetration (usually 0.6 mm). The device is pressed against the skin in a similar fashion to derma-stamps, but the product stored in the attached vial can flow down the needles and into the newly created micro-channels in the skin.

- *Plasma shower:* Plasma is an ionised gas with electrical energy. A strong low-temperature atmospheric plasma on the surface of the skin both sterilises the skin and increases the absorption rate by temporarily breaking the cell adhesion molecules (CAMs) that connect the skin cells, effectively enabling a transdermal drug delivery system of certain products applied topically.

- *'No needle' injector:* Jet injection devices have already been used as an insulin delivery method for diabetics, but recently the technology has filtered through to the aesthetics industry as a 'needle-free' alternative for intradermal, subcutaneous, and intramuscular product delivery. Devices are usually either composed of a disposable sterile cartridge inside a casing activated by a spring-push mechanism with product delivered into the skin mechanically using high air pressure or by a low-pressure gas cylinder driven system. For mesotherapy products, this may be a safe and valid route of administration. However, there is currently insufficient data on safety and efficacy of products such as cross-linked HA at the time of writing for any further recommendations to be made.

The most common areas of treatment include the face and neck, but mesotherapy can also be used for the décolletage, hands, arms, knees, and abdominal area.

The skin quality market is a rapidly expanding one, with numerous products aiming to improve skin appearances. As the term 'mesotherapy' covers a wide range of treatments with different goals and results, we will divide the products used in mesotherapy into four broad categories:

- Skin boosters
- Bio-stimulators
- Growth factors
- PRP

Skin Boosters

Example products include Redensity 1 (Teoxane), Restylane Vital (Galderma), RRS (Aesthetic Dermal), Viscoderm Skinko/Skinko E/Hydrobooster (IBSA Italia), Volite (Allergan), Definisse Hydrobooster (Relife), NCTF-HA135 (FillMed), and Sunekos (Professional Dietetics).

How Does It Work?

Skin boosters all vary slightly in their 'cocktail' mix, but in general consist of a combination of HA, minerals, amino acids, and vitamins. Unlike traditional HA fillers, these are either non-cross-linked, or only very slightly cross-linked, HA. This means that the HA is more 'free' to spread under the skin, rather than being held together in a clump by the cross-linking. As the HA molecules can hold up to 1000 times their own weight in water, this provides a hydrating effect to the skin as they spread, without causing significant volumisation to the area injected.

It has also been demonstrated that HA alone, or combined with vitamin 'cocktails', helps maintain skin fibroblast cell proliferation [59], and that intradermal injection can stimulate production of new undamaged collagen [60]. Due to the non-cross-linked or non-stabilised nature of the HA in most of these products, it does not remain in the skin as long compared with cross-linked/stabilised HA (less than 24 hours [61]).

The addition of minerals, amino acids, and vitamins all act as 'nutrients' for the skin, helping to improve and maintain cellular trophism of the epidermis and papillary dermis, acting on the fibroblast and keratinocytes. The deep action on fibroblasts helps maintain/improve skin elasticity, while the superficial action on keratinocytes improves the protective barrier from external damage (dermal thickness).

The treatments tend to consist of 1–4 treatments, with 1–3 weeks between each session. Results tend to last, on average, around 6 months.

Who Is a Suitable Candidate?

The ideal patients are those who:

- Require improvement to skin hydration and quality
- Would benefit from some thickening of the skin
- Are scared to go down the filler and/or botulinum toxin route
- Wish to target fine lines

What Are the Benefits?

Treatments can be used in all adult age ranges – those on the younger side of the scale may like the brightening effect on their skin that these treatments can achieve, and to help to create a fresh 'dewy glow', whilst the more mature patients appreciate the extra hydration, skin scaffolding support, and fine wrinkle improvements.

What Are the Limitations?

- Skin boosters are not suitable for replacing significant volume loss.
- A greater time commitment is usually required to complete the course.
- Downtime can vary. In general, the products disperse within the skin very quickly and any blebs are usually not visible after 24 hours, but as with any injectable, bruising is a definite risk and something to plan carefully with the patient due to the repeat treatments they will require to complete the course.

Pearls of Wisdom

These can be a great tool to have in treating tricky areas like the periorbital region and 'necklace lines'.

Bio-Stimulators

Profhilo (IBSA Italia) is a great example of bio-stimulators.

How Does It Work?

As previously mentioned, decreased fibroblast activity is one of the primary skin ageing processes, as this leads to a reduction in the biosynthesis of dermal extracellular matrix components and HA, resulting in loss of skin elasticity and turgidity [62, 63].

Bio-stimulators aim to improve skin quality, texture, laxity, and hydration by supporting keratinocyte, fibroblast and adipocyte viability, leading to a remodelling of the extracellular matrix in terms of elasticity and support. The bio-stimulator within this category contains a mix of high (H-HA) and low (L-HA) molecular weight HA. L-HA is regenerative in nature, binding to specific receptors and stimulating fibroblasts and keratinocyte proliferation. This provides nourishment and deep hydration to the aged skin [64], stimulates elastin and four different types of collagen (types I and III in fibroblasts, types IV and VII in keratinocytes) [65] for improved tissue remodelling. H-HA, owing to its high capacity to bind water molecules and interact with collagen and proteoglycans, exerts a dermal scaffold action for a volumetric effect.

Bio-stimulators generally do not create substantial volume at one specific point when compared with fillers – rather, once injected, the product will spread smoothly underneath the skin to form a larger area of stimulation. Bio-stimulators would therefore be the incorrect choice for sculpting projected contours and angles, for example, in cheekbones and jawlines.

Who Is a Suitable Candidate?

- Those with dehydrated, dull, and/or photoaged skin.
- Patients aged between 40 and 60 will have the most noticeable improvement. However, as adults lose 1% of collagen per year [66], this could be considered as a preventative treatment in younger patients.
- Patients demonstrating crêpey skin texture.
- Mild sagging/laxity of the skin.

What Are the Benefits?

As well as providing hydration, bio-stimulators have a greater tightening/lifting effect when compared with products such as skin boosters. As the L-HA and H-HA chains are thermally stabilised together, the HA is more slowly released into the skin over approximately 28 days, allowing a greater level of stimulation compared with non-stabilised HA. Without this stabilisation, HA would break down within 24 hours [61]. This is also a chemical-free method of stabilisation, compared with the BDDE (1,4-butanediol diglycidyl ether) chemical cross-linking used in some volumising fillers.

What Are the Limitations?

- Bio-stimulators are not suitable for revolumisation
- Manual injections have to be performed at the intradermal level
- Risk of bruising
- A course of multiple sessions is required for optimum result

Pearls of Wisdom

When treating crêpey necks (a traditionally difficult area to treat), bio-stimulators can be a good first-line treatment. In those with greater volume loss, fillers can also be used as an adjunct.

Growth Factors

Example products include AQ Growth Factors (AQ Skin Solutions), Calecim Professional Serum, Endocare Growth Factor (AesthetiCare), and SkinGenuity.

How Does It Work?

Growth factors and cytokines are naturally occurring substances – usually proteins or hormones – which act as signalling molecules that bind to specific receptors on the surface of their target cells and induce signalling pathways. These can regulate an array of biological processes [67]; however, of particular interest in aesthetics is the involvement in cell differentiation, angiogenesis, production and distribution of collagen and elastin, and the regulation of essential cellular activities – the outcome of which can support healthy skin structure and function by promoting cell growth and recovery, as well as organising the extracellular matrix [68]. Put simply, by replacing or helping to regenerate the cells that the body loses in the natural ageing process, such as collagen, fibrin, and elastin, we can help treat ageing skin. Examples include insulin-like growth factor (IGF), epidermal growth factor (EGF), transforming growth factor (TGF), and fibroblast growth factor (FGF) [69]. Cytokines are closely related to growth factors, and often the two terms are used interchangeably – the distinction between them is frequently arbitrary and stems more from the manner of their discovery rather than from a clear difference in function. For the purposes of this chapter, we shall refer to both as simply growth factors (GFs).

Often, for best/optimal results, products with a selection of several different GF result in best outcome. This is because of the different functions that act on different cell types. Solutions of single growth factor products do not supply the variety of signalling to induce the correct combined effects of growth, proliferation, differentiation, healing and inhibition of inflammatory cytokines [70].

Who Is a Suitable Candidate?

Patients with evidence of photo-damaged skin, hair loss/thinning, visible effects of chronological ageing, and premature ageing due to environmental factors.

What Are the Benefits?

- Proliferation of blood vessels, thereby increasing nutrient and oxygen delivery to tissues
- Neocollagenesis
- Relatively painless treatment with microneedling
- No downtime

What Are the Limitations?

- Growth factors are large molecules, which limits their ability to pass into the skin unaided.
- If solely applied topically, they can only pass through hair follicles, sweat glands, or by chemical modification with lipophilic molecules [71].
- A course of treatments is required for optimum result.
- May take time for results to show.

Pearls of Wisdom

Due to their anti-inflammatory effects, growth factors can help to reduce downtime in the days after laser resurfacing, microneedling, plasma blepharoplasty, and other invasive skin treatments when applied post-procedure.

Platelet-Rich Plasma (PRP)

Now that we have a basic understanding of growth factors, we can better appreciate the basis of PRP treatment in aesthetics.

How Does It Work?

PRP is defined as 'a volume of autologous plasma that has a platelet concentration above baseline' [72]. These platelets, once activated, secrete several different growth factors which work to stimulate tissue regeneration by cell proliferation, angiogenesis, tissue remodelling, and inflammatory responses, inducing the synthesis of new collagen by fibroblasts [73].

In order to create PRP, a sample of blood is extracted from the patient into a tube with anticoagulant, placed in a centrifuge and spun to separate the plasma according to the differing densities of the components – red blood cells being the heaviest layer at the bottom, a middle layer of white blood cells and platelets (the buffy coat, platelet rich), followed by a plasma layer (platelet poor) on top. These top two layers are then extracted to form 'PRP', which can then be activated and injected back into the patient.

Activation is required in order to release the growth factors from the platelets. PRP can be activated exogenously by thrombin, calcium chloride, or mechanical trauma [74]. Collagen is also a natural activator of PRP, thus when PRP is used in soft tissue, it can be argued that it does not necessarily need to be exogenously activated.

Another important variable is that the concentration of platelets within PRP generally varies from 2.5 to 9 times above baseline between different manufacturers [75], and there is currently no standardised consensus on the optimal value. While it may seem logical that plasma with the highest possible platelet concentration will get better results than plasma with a lower platelet concentration, that is not necessarily the case. One lab study suggested that plasma with concentrations 2.5 times that of normal blood was ideal [76], and others have found higher concentrations might actually limit new cell growth [77].

Who Is a Suitable Candidate?

Patients with evidence of photo-damaged skin, visible effects of chronological ageing, hair loss/thinning, premature ageing due to environmental factors, and acne scarring.

What Are the Benefits?

- Autologous
- No risk of allergic/sensitivity reaction
- Considered a more natural approach to skin rejuvenation

What Are the Limitations?

Results may vary according to preparation techniques and patient's general health – those with a healthy lifestyle tend to have healthier platelets and therefore get better results. It is important to note that due to the fluidity of PRP, it is unsuitable for revolumisation and/or dermal augmentation, and only remains within the tissue for approximately 48 hours [78] due to early washout [79]. Platelet-rich fibrin (PRF) may be better suited for this purpose, but this is beyond the scope of this chapter. A course of three treatments, a month apart, is usually advised as a starting point.

Pearls of Wisdom

- A useful adjunct to consider for treating periorbital 'dark circles' in cases where this is caused by thin/translucent skin.
- As with growth factors, PRP can be used in conjunction with other treatments to aid in faster recovery between treatments.

Conclusion

Healthy skin texture should be smooth, evenly pigmented, well hydrated and overlying a well-supported dermis. Unfortunately, there is no quick fix to achieving optimal skin texture; a patient must be committed to an ongoing skincare regime tailored to their individual skin needs.

Skin deep beauty is something we can now address as aesthetic practitioners; the person's character, however, is entirely up to the patient!

REFERENCES

1. Kolarsick PAJ, Kolarsick MA, Goodwin C, "Anatomy and physiology of the skin," *Journal of the Dermatology Nurses Association*, vol. 3, no. 4, pp. 203–213, 2011.
2. Anatomy of the Skin. Johns Hopkins Medicine. Accessed online on 27 January 2019: https://www.hopkinsmedicine.org/healthlibrary/conditions/dermatology/anatomy_of_the_skin_85,P01336.
3. Gilchrest BA, "Photoaging," *Journal of Investigative Dermatology*, vol. 133, no. E1, pp. E2–E6, 2013.
4. Chung JH, Seo JY, Choi HR, et al. "Modulation of skin collagen metabolism in aged and photoaged human skin in vivo," *Journal of Investigative Dermatology*, vol. 117, no. 5, pp. 1218–1224, 2001.
5. Talwar HS, Griffiths CE, Fisher GJ, Hamilton TA, Voorhees JJ, "Reduced type I and type III procollagens in photodamaged adult human skin," *Journal of Investigative Dermatology*, vol. 105, no. 2, pp. 285–290, 1995.
6. Valacchi G, Sticozzi C, Pecorelli A, Cervallati F, Cervallati C, Maioli E, "Cutaneous responses to environmental stressors," *Annals of the New York Academy of Sciences*, vol. 1271, pp. 75–81, 2012.
7. Uitto J, "The role of elastin and collagen in cutaneous aging: Intrinsic aging versus photoexposure," *Journal of Drugs in Dermatology*, vol. 7, 2 Suppl, pp. s12–s16, 2008.
8. Weihermann AC, Lorencini M, Brohem CA, de Carvalho CM, "Elastin structure and its involvement in skin photoageing," *International Journal of Cosmetic Science*, vol. 39, no. 3, pp. 241–247, 2017.
9. Papakonstantinou E, Roth M, Karakiulakis G, "Hyaluronic acid: A key molecule in skin aging," *Dermatoendocrinology*, vol. 4, no. 3, pp. 253–258, 2012.
10. Oliveira Gonzalez AC, Costa TF, Andrade ZA, Medrado AR, "Wound healing – A literature review," *Anais Brasileiros de Dermatologia*, vol. 91, no. 5, pp. 614–620, 2016.
11. Stamford NPJ, "Stability, transdermal penetration, and cutaneous effects of ascorbic acid and its derivatives," *Journal of Cosmetic Dermatology*, vol. 11, no. 4, 310–317, 2012.
12. Joshua Zeichner, quoted in Kinonen S, Wirt S, Hoshikawa K. The Best Vitamin C Serums, Moisturizers, and More for Brighter Skin. Allure 2020: https://www.allure.com/gallery/get-brighter-skin-vitamin-c.
13. Susie Wang, quoted in Nims B. What the Heck Does Vitamin C Serum Do for Your Skin, Anyway? Huffington Post 2019: https://www.huffingtonpost.co.uk/entry/what-does-vitamin-cserum-do-for-the-skin.

14. Telang PS, "Vitamin C in dermatology," *Indian Dermatology Online Journal*, vol. 4, no. 2, pp. 143–146, 2013.
15. Amanda von dem Hagen, quoted in Wida EC. What Is Retinol? Here Are the Benefits, Uses and Side Effects You Need to Know. *Today* 2019: https://www.today.com/style/what-retinol-retinolbenefits-uses-side-effects-more-t150639.
16. Murad H, The Science behind Retinol (Vitamin A). Happi 2012: https://www.happi.com/issues/2012-03/view_experts-opinion/thescience-behind-retinol-vitamin-a/.
17. Ursin F, Steger F, Borelli C, "Katharsis of the skin: Peeling applications and agents of chemical peelings in Greek medical textbooks of Graeco-Roman antiquity," *Journal of the European Academy of Dermatology and Venereology*, vol. 32, no. 11, pp. 2034–2040, 2018.
18. Loretta Ciraldo, in Brucculleri J. What Does Glycolic Acid Do for Your Skin? Dermatologists Explain. Huffington Post 2018: https://www.huffingtonpost.co.uk/entry/what-is-glycolicacid_n_5b68706ae4b0d e86f4a3cf8e.
19. Irwin B, TCA Peels – Frequently Asked Questions. SkinTour [accessed Dec 2020]: https://www.skintour.com/face-focus/peels-and-microdermabrasion/tca-peels/.
20. Brannon HL, The History of Microdermabrasion. VeryWellHealth 2020: https://www.verywellhealth.com/the-history-of-microdermabrasion-1069228.
21. Stamatina G, Sotiris TG, Aglaia V, "Plexr in acne treatment," *Pinnacle Medicine & Medical Sciences*, vol. 2, no. 1, pp. 1–5, 2015.
22. Heinlin J, Morfill G, Landthaler M, et al. "Plasma medicine: Possible applications in dermatology," *Journal of the German Society of Dermatology*, vol. 8, no. 12, pp. 968–976, 2010.
23. Bernhardt T, Semele ML, Schäfer M, Bekeschus S, Emmert S, Boeckmann L, "Plasma medicine: Applications of cold atmospheric pressure plasma in dermatology," *Oxidative Medicine and Cellular Longevity,*, 3873928, 2019. doi: 10.1155/2019/3873928.
24. Crofford R, "A review of plasma medicine," *PMFA Journal*, vol. 6, no. 3, 2019.
25. Pourazizi M, Abraham-Naeini B, "Plasma application in aesthetic medicine: Clinical and physical aspects," *Journal of Surgical Dermatology*, vol. 2, no. T1, 2017.
26. Gloustianou G, Safari M, Tsioumas S, Vlachodimitropoulos, Scarano A, "Presentation of old and new histological results after plasma exercises (plexr) application (regeneration of the skin tissue with collagen III)," *Pinnacle Medicine & Medical Sciences*, vol. 3, pp. 983–990, 2016.
27. Rossi E, Farnetani F, Trakatelli M, Ciardo S, Pellacani G, "Clinical and confocal microscopy study of plasma exeresis for non-surgical blepharoplasty of the upper eyelid: A pilot study," *Dermatologic Surgery*, vol. 44, no. 2, pp. 283–290, 2018.
28. King M, "Focus on plasma: The application of plasma devices in aesthetic medicine," *PMFA Journal*, vol. 5, no. 5, pp. 24–26, 2017.
29. Anderson A, Special Feature: Lasers and Lights. Aesthetics 2015: http://aesthetics journal.com/feature/lasers-and-lights.
30. Anderson RR, Parrish JA, "Selective photothermolysis: Precise microsurgery by selective absorption of pulsed radiation," *Science*, vol. 220, pp. 524–527, 1983.
31. Trivedi MK, Yang FC, Cho BK, "A review of laser and light therapy in melasma," *International Journal of Women's Dermatology*, vol. 3, no. 1, pp. 11–20, 2017.
32. Li YH, Chen JZS, Wei HC, et al. "Efficacy and safety of intense pulsed light in treatment of melasma in Chinese patients," *Dermatologic Surgery*, vol. 34, pp. 693–701, 2008.
33. Goldman M, "One laser for a cosmetic/dermatologic practice," *The Journal of Clinical and Aesthetic Dermatology*, vol. 4, no. 5, pp. 18–21, 2011.
34. Pai GS, Pai AH, "Q switched laser treatment for freckles in individuals with skin type V," *Aesthetics in Dermatology and Surgery*, vol. 1, pp. 2–7, 2017.
35. Choi JE, Lee DW, Seo SH, Ahn HH, Kye YC, "Low fluence Q-switched Nd:YAG laser for the treatment of melasma in Asian patients," *Journal of Cosmetic Dermatology*, vo. 17, no. 6, pp. 1053–1058, 2018.
36. Omi T, Neumann K, "The role of the CO_2 laser and fractional CO_2 laser in dermatology," *Laser Therapy*, vol. 23, no. 1, pp. 49–60, 2014.
37. Saki N, "Picosecond laser applications in aesthetic dermatology," *Journal of Aesthetic Surgical Dermatology*, vol. 2, no. T1, 2017.
38. Ramsell WM, "Fractional CO_2 laser resurfacing complications," *Seminars in Plastic Surgery*, vol. 26, no. 3, pp. 137–140, 2012.

39. Sklar LR, Burnett CT, Waibel JS, Moy RL, Ozog DM, "Laser assisted drug delivery: A review of an evolving technology," *Lasers in Surgery and Medicine*, vol. 46, no. 4, pp. 249–262, 2014.

40. White WM, Makin IRS, Barthe PG, Slayton MH, Gliklich RE, "Selective creation of thermal injury zones in the superficial musculoaponeurotic system using intense ultrasound therapy: A new target for non invasive facial rejuvenation," *Archives of Facial Plastic Surgery*, vol. 9, pp. 22–29, 2007.

41. Brobst RW, Ferguson M, Perkins SW, "Ulthera: Initial and six month results," *Facial Plastic Surgery Clinics of North America*, vol. 20, pp. 163–176, 2012.

42. Nassab R, "The evidence behind non-invasive body contouring devices," *Aesthetic Surgery Journal*, vol. 35, no. 3, pp. 279–293, 2015.

43. Kharki A, Kisyova R, "High intensity focused ultrasound (HIFU) technology for body contouring," *Journal of Aesthetic Nursing*, Suppl 1, 2019.

44. Jewell ML, Baxter RA, Cox SE, et al. "Randomised sham controlled trial to evaluate the safety and effectiveness of a high-intensity focused ultrasound device for non invasive body sculpting," *Plastic and Reconstructive Surgery*, vol. 128, no. I, pp. 253–262, 2011.

45. Park H, Kim E, Kim J, Ro Y, Ko J, "High-intensity focused ultrasound for the treatment of wrinkles and skin laxity in seven different facial areas," *Annals of Dermatology*, vol. 27, no. 6, pp. 688–693, 2015.

46. Kaminaka C, Furukawa F, Yamamoto Y, "Long term clinical and histological effects of a bipolar fractional radiofrequency system in the treatment of facial atrophic acne scars and acne vulgaris in Japanese patients: A series of eight cases," *Photo Medicine and Laser Surgery*, vol. 34, pp. 656–660, 2016.

47. Lolis MS, Goldberg DJ, "Radiofrequency in cosmetic dermatology: A review," *Dermatologic Surgery*, pp. 1765–1776, 2012.

48. Sadick NS, Nassar AH, Dorizas AS, Alexiades-Armenakas M, "Bipolar and multipolar radiofrequency," *Dermatologic Surgery*, Suppl 12, pp. S174–S179, 2014.

49. Royo de la torre J, Moreno-Moraga J, Muñoz E, Navarro PC, *The Journal of Clinical and Aesthetic Dermatology*, vol. 4, no. 1, pp. 28–35, 2011.

50. Görgü M, Gökkaya A, Kizilkan J, Karanfil E, Dogan A, "Rafiofrequency: Review of the literature," *Turkish Journal of Plastic Surgery*, vol. 27, pp. 62–72, 2019.

51. Fistonić I, Sorta Bilajac Turin's I, Fistonić N, Marton I, "Short term efficacy and safety of focused monopolar radiofrequency device for labial laxity improvement – noninvasive labia tissue tightening. A prospective cohort study," *Lasers in Surgery and Medicine*, vol. 48, pp. 254–259, 2016.

52. de Felipe I, Del Cueto SR, Perez E, Redondo P, "Adverse reactions after nonablative radiofrequency: Follow-up of 290 patients," *Journal of Cosmetic Dermatology*, vol. 6, no. 3, pp. 63–66, 2007.

53. Cambridge Dictionary [Internet] Cambridge University Press; 2020. Beauty is only skin deep; [cited 2020 Apr 15]; available from https://dictionary.cambridge.org/dictionary/english/beauty-is-only-skin-deep.

54. Fink B, Grammer K, Matts P, "Visible skin color distribution plays a role in the perception of age, attractiveness, and health in female faces," *Evolution and Human Behavior*, vol. 27, no. 6, pp. 433–442, 2006.

55. Fink B, Matts P, D'Emiliano D, Bunse L, Weege B, Röder S, "Colour homogeneity and visual perception of age, health and attractiveness of male facial skin," *Journal of European Academy of Dermatology and Venereology*, vol. 26, no. 12, pp. 1486–1492, 2012.

56. Dalens M, Prikhnenko S, "Polycomponent mesotherapy formulations for the treatment of skin aging and improvement of skin quality," *Clinical, Cosmetic and Investigational Dermatology*, vol. 151, 2015.

57. Iorizzo M, De Padova M, Tosti A, "Biorejuvenation: Theory and practice," *Clinics in Dermatology*, vol. 26, no. 2, pp. 177–181, 2008.

58. Iriarte C, Awosika O, Rengifo-Pardo M, Ehrlich A, "Review of applications of microneedling in dermatology," *Clinical, Cosmetic and Investigational Dermatology*, vol. 10, pp. 289–298, 2017.

59. Jäger C, Brenner C, Habicht J, Wallich R, "Bioactive reagents used in mesotherapy for skin rejuvenation in vivo induce diverse physiological processes in human skin fibroblasts in vitro – A pilot study," *Experimental Dermatology*, vol. 21, no. 1, pp. 72–75, 2011.

60. Quan T, Wang F, Shao Y, et al. "Enhancing structural support of the dermal microenvironment activates fibroblasts, endothelial cells, and deratinocytes in aged human skin in vivo," *Journal of Investigative Dermatology*, vol. 133, no. 3, pp. 658–667, 2013.

61. Matarasso S, Carruthers J, Jewell M, "Consensus recommendations for soft-tissue augmentation with nonanimal stabilized hyaluronic acid (restylane)," *Plastic and Reconstructive Surgery*, vol. 117, Suppl, pp. 3S–34S, 2006.

62. Zimbler MS, Kokoska MS, Thomas JR, "Anatomy and pathophysiology of facial aging," *Facial Plastic Surgery Clinics of North America*, vol. 9, no. 2, pp. 179–187, 2001.

63. Ghersetich I, Lotti T, Campanile G, Grappone C, Dini G, "Hyaluronic acid in cutaneous intrinsic aging," *International Journal of Dermatology*, vol. 33, no. 2, pp. 119–122, 1994.

64. D'Agostino A, Stellavato A, Busico T, et al. "In vitro analysis of the effects on wound healing of high- and low-molecular weight chains of hyaluronan and their hybrid H-HA/L-HA complexes," *BMC Molecular and Cell Biology*, vol. 16, no. 1, 2015.

65. Stellavato A, Corsuto L, D'Agostino A, et al. "Hyaluronan hybrid cooperative complexes as a novel frontier for cellular bioprocesses re-activation," *PLOS One*, vol. 11, no. 10, 2016.

66. Shuster S, Black M, Mcvitie E, "The influence of age and sex on skin thickness, skin collagen and density," *British Journal of Dermatology*, vol. 93, no. 6, pp. 639–643, 1975.

67. Wilson J, Hunt T, *Molecular Biology of the Cell*, 4th ed. New York, NY: Garland Science; 2002.

68. Schuldiner M, Yanuka O, Itskovitz-Eldor J, Melton D, Benvenisty N, "Effects of eight growth factors on the differentiation of cells derived from human embryonic stem cells," *Proceedings of the National Academy of Sciences of United States of America*, vol. 97, no. 21, pp. 11307–11312, 2000.

69. Bafinco A, Aaronson S, *Classification of Growth Factors and Their Receptors. Cancer Medicine 6.* Hamilton, Ontario: BC Decker; 2003.

70. Barrientos S, Stojadinovic O, Golinko M, Brem H, Tomic-Canic M, "Perspective article: Growth factors and cytokines in wound healing," *Wound Repair and Regeneration*, vol. 16, no. 5, pp. 585–601, 2008.

71. Schaefer H, Lademann J, "The role of follicular penetration," *Skin Pharmacology and Physiology*, vol. 14, no. 1, pp. 23–27, 2001.

72. Marx R, "Platelet-rich plasma (PRP): What is PRP and what is not PRP?" *Implant Dentistry*, vol. 10, no. 4, pp. 225–228, 2001.

73. Kim D, Je Y, Kim C, et al. "Can platelet-rich plasma be used for skin rejuvenation? Evaluation of effects of platelet-rich plasma on human dermal fibroblast," *Annals of Dermatology*, vol. 23, no. 4, p. 424, 2011.

74. Marlovits S, Mousavi M, Gäbler C, Erdös J, Vécsei V, "A new simplified technique for producing platelet-rich plasma: a short technical note," *European Spine Journal*, vol. 13, no. S01, pp. S102–S106, 2004.

75. ECRI Institute. AHRQ Healthcare Horizon Scanning System Potential High Impact Interventions: Priority Area 01: Arthritis and Nontraumatic Joint Disease. (Prepared by ECRI Institute under Contract No. HHSA290201000006C.) Rockville, MD: Agency for Healthcare Research and Quality. June 2013. effectivehealthcare.ahrq.gov.

76. Rughetti A, Giusti I, D'Ascenzo S, et al. "Platelet gel-released supernatant modulates the angiogenic capability of human endothelial cells," *Blood Transfusion*, vol. 6, pp. 12–17, 2008.

77. Graziani F, Ivanovski S, Cei S, Ducci F, Tonetti M, Gabriele M, "The in vitro effect of different PRP concentrations on osteoblasts and fibroblasts," *Clinical Oral Implants Research*, vol. 17, no. 2, pp. 212–219, 2006.

78. Sclafani A. "Safety, efficacy, and utility of platelet-rich fibrin matrix in facial plasticsurgery," *Archives of Facial Plastic Surgery*, vol. 13, no. 4, 247, 2011.

79. Matz E, Pearlman A, Terlecki R, "Safety and feasibility of platelet rich fibrin matrix injections for treatment of common urologic conditions," *Investigative and Clinical Urology*, vol. 59, no. 1, p. 61, 2018.

3

The Forehead

Vincent Wong

CONTENTS

The forehead forms the upper third of the face. The hairline marks the top of the forehead and the supraorbital ridge defines the bottom margin. The supraorbital ridge, which is more prominent in males, is the bony structure situated above the eyes (overlaid by eyebrows) that separates the forehead from the mid-face. The sides of the forehead are characterised by the temporal ridges, situated on the sides of the face [1, 2]. See Figure 3.1.

Horizontal Wrinkles

Horizontal wrinkles on the forehead are produced by contractions of the frontalis muscle. The frontalis muscle is responsible for raising the brows and plays a major role in facial expressions. Individuals who tend to express their emotions through facial expressions will have more frequent contractions throughout their life. Those with upper eyelid ptosis would experience constant contraction of frontalis

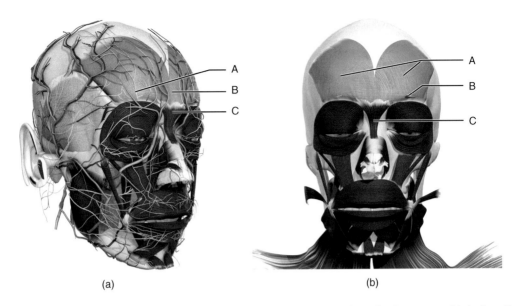

(a)   (b)

FIGURE 3.1 Muscles affecting the forehead. (a) A, corrugator supercilii; B, frontalis; C, procerus. (b) A, frontalis; B, corrugator supercilii; C, procerus. (Adapted from www.anatomy.tv with permission © Informa UK Ltd [trading as Primal Pictures], 2021.)

as a compensation mechanism to keep the eyes open and visual field clear. These, in turn, will result in a more active muscle leading to deeper horizontal wrinkles across the forehead due to increased muscle tone. There are two types of wrinkles, namely dynamic (wrinkles that come on during facial expression) and static wrinkles (those that are present even when the face is at rest).

Rating Scales

Severity of forehead wrinkles can be assessed using the scales in Figure 3.2.

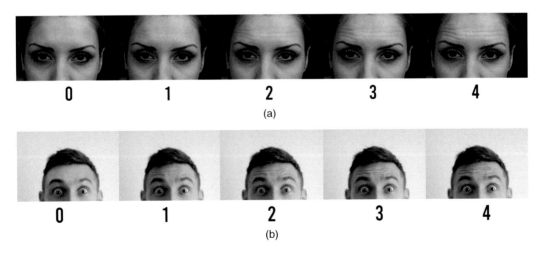

FIGURE 3.2 (a) Horizontal forehead wrinkle assessment scale at rest. (b) Horizontal forehead wrinkle assessment on animation (raising eyebrows). 0 = no wrinkle, 1 = mild wrinkles, 2 = moderate wrinkles, 3 = severe wrinkles, 4 = very severe wrinkles (following the scales of Merz Aesthetics).

Treatment Options

- Neurotoxin

    Neurotoxin (botulinum toxin type A) works by inhibiting the release of the neurotransmitter acetylcholine from motor nerve endings. In order for muscle contraction to occur, the acetylcholine must be released from its vesicle, through the neuromuscular junction, to the end-plate region.

    Neurotoxin initially binds to special receptors on the external membranes of motor cholinergic neurons and exists as a heavy chain and a light chain attached by a disulphide bond. Endocytosis then occurs, and the neurotoxin particle forms a vesicle in the motor neuron terminal. The bond between the chains is then broken; the light chain enters the cytoplasm and splits the protein SNAP-25 (Synaptosomal-Associated Protein) needed for the SNARE (SNAP Receptors) complex formation [3]. This then inhibits exocytosis of vesicles containing acetylcholine so muscle contractions are inhibited, making neurotoxin an effective treatment for dynamic wrinkles.

    Neurotoxin is injected intramuscularly into the frontalis muscle in the forehead. As the frontalis muscle is the only eyebrow elevator, care must be taken to ensure that injections are 3 cm above the eyebrows to prevent eyebrow ptosis. Generally, 10–15 standardised units of neurotoxin are sufficient, although male patients and those with taller forehead or receding hairline may require a higher dose to achieve aesthetically pleasing results:

- Dermal filler

    With prolonged muscle contractions and age, some patients may find that wrinkles are not only present when making an expression but also when they are relaxed. For these static lines in the forehead, hyaluronic acid dermal filler could be an option (preferably after neurotoxin treatment) as it has the ability to restore lost volume in the region, giving a fresh and supple appearance. When injected into the forehead, dermal fillers can also increase collagen production in the area temporarily. A low-viscosity, cross-linked dermal filler can be injected along the static wrinkles (in the dermis) to restore volume in the area. Care must be taken when injecting fillers in the forehead due to the vascularity of the region.

Combination Treatments

- Combination of neurotoxin and dermal fillers
- Skin peel
- Mesotherapy
- Laser treatments
- Platelet-rich plasma

Complications

- Oedema (from needle trauma)
- Bruising (from needle trauma)
- Vascular compromise (from dermal filler injections)
- Necrosis (from dermal filler blocking an artery)
- Eyebrow ptosis (from paralysing inferior fibres of frontalis)
- Infection (from lack of aseptic technique)

Vertical Wrinkles

Vertical frown lines are produced predominantly by contractions of two muscles, the procerus and the corrugator supercilii. The product of the joint contractions of these muscles gives the appearance of a frown, which can make an individual look unhappy and angry. The procerus runs vertically and is

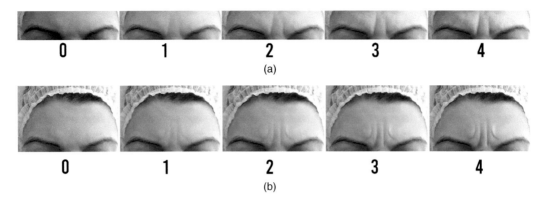

FIGURE 3.3   (a) Glabella wrinkle assessment scale at rest. (b) Glabella wrinkle assessment on animation (frowning). 0 = no wrinkle, 1 = mild wrinkles, 2 = moderate wrinkles, 3 = severe wrinkles, 4 = very severe wrinkles (following the scales of Merz Aesthetics).

located in between the eyebrows. When active, it produces folds and bunching of skin across the bridge of the nose. The creasing of the skin along the eyebrows that brings them closer together is a result of the contraction of the corrugator supercilia muscles. Similar to wrinkles created by the frontalis, overuse of these muscles through ageing and environmental factors will lead to deeper wrinkles on the forehead.

Rating Scales

Severity of glabella wrinkles can be assessed using the scale in Figure 3.3.

Treatment Options

- Neurotoxin

  Similar to horizontal lines, neurotoxin injections can produce great results in this region. An average dose of 15–25 units of neurotoxin is usually required. It is important to inject deeply in the procerus and medial parts of the corrugator muscle, while keeping injections in the lateral parts of corrugator superficial to achieve best results. All injections should be at least 1 cm away from the orbital rim.

- Dermal filler

  A low-viscosity, cross-linked dermal filler can be injected along the static wrinkles (in the dermis) to restore volume in the glabella (preferably after neurotoxin treatment). Extra care must be taken when injecting fillers in this region due to the number of small superficial vessels.

Combination Treatments

- Combination of neurotoxin and dermal fillers
- Skin peel
- Mesotherapy
- Laser treatments
- Platelet-rich plasma

Complications

- Oedema (from needle trauma)
- Bruising (from needle trauma)
- Vascular compromise (from dermal filler injections)

- Necrosis (from dermal filler blocking an artery)
- Infection (from lack of aseptic technique)

Volume Loss and Reshaping

A full forehead without obvious supraorbital bossing is the characteristic of a female face, whereas a slight concavity in the forehead with prominent supraorbital bossing is considered to be masculine. In certain cultures, a full forehead is also a sign of prosperity. Chronological ageing can lead to volume loss in the forehead, especially with muscle atrophy. Patients who want more feminine features may also consider forehead volumisation treatments.

Treatment Option

- Dermal filler

  Dermal fillers are commonly injected in the forehead to replace lost volume or to reshape the region. This can be achieved with a 27G needle or 25G cannula, with dermal filler placement in the supraperiosteal level. Extra care must be taken to avoid important vessels (supratrochlear artery in central forehead, supraorbital artery in medial forehead, and superficial temporal artery in lateral forehead).

- Autologous fat

Autologous fat transfer can also be used to revolumise the forehead, in a similar way to dermal fillers. The key differences between dermal fillers and autologous fat are covered in Chapter 11.

Combination Treatments

- Combination of neurotoxin and dermal fillers
- Skin peel
- Mesotherapy
- Laser treatments
- Platelet-rich plasma

Complications

- Oedema (from needle trauma)
- Bruising (from needle trauma)
- Vascular compromise
- Necrosis
- Infection (from lack of aseptic technique)

Case Study 3.1

Patient Age: 32
  Sex: Male

Presenting Concern

- Static forehead and glabella wrinkles, but wants to maintain facial movements in these areas (top photo of Figure 3.4)

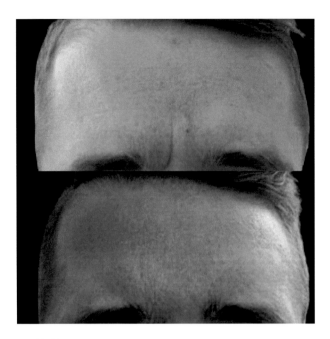

FIGURE 3.4   Patient: top and bottom.

Grading (before)

- *Glabella*: Grade 3 (severe)
- *Forehead*: Grade 2 (mild)

Treatment Plan

- *Session 1*: Botulinum toxin using Botox by Allergan (25 units to glabella, 10 units to forehead) (Figure 3.5)

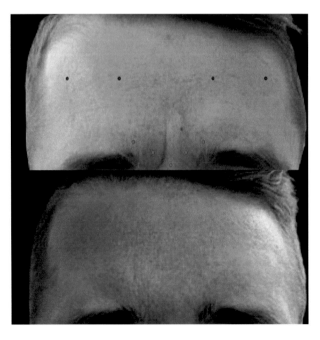

FIGURE 3.5   Blue dots, 5 u Botox per injection; red dots, 2.5 u Botox per injection.

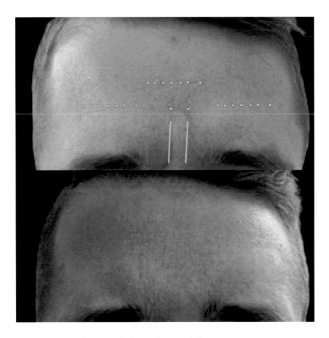

FIGURE 3.6 Straight lines, retrograde linear technique; dots, serial puncture.

- *Session 2*: Dermal filler using Definisse Touch by Relife (1 ml used in total) (Figure 3.6)
- *Session 3*: Superficial skin peel using Obagi Blu-Peel Radiance (Figure 3.7)

Grading (after)

- *Glabella*: Grade 0 (none)
- *Forehead*: Grade 0 (none)

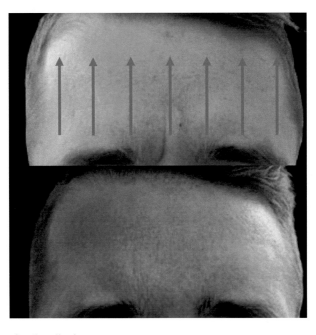

FIGURE 3.7 Direction of peel application.

Case Study 3.2

Patient Age: 49
  Sex: Female

Presenting Concern

- Dynamic horizontal wrinkles in the forehead, but would like to maintain some forehead movement.

Grading (before)

- 3 (severe) (Figure 3.8)

Treatment Plan

- Botulinum toxin using Botox by Allergan (10 units to forehead) (Figure 3.9)

Grading (after)

- *Forehead*: Grade 0 (none)

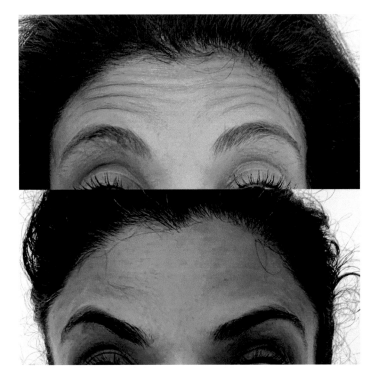

FIGURE 3.8   Patient: top and bottom.

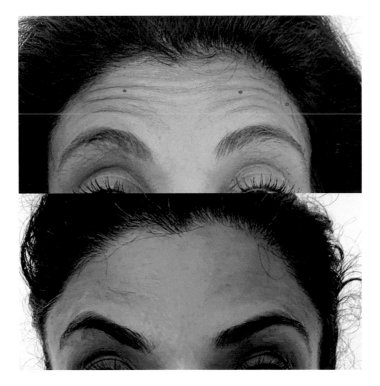

FIGURE 3.9 Blue dot, 2.5 u of Botox.

REFERENCES

1. Medical website. Forehead Anatomy. Accessed online on 5 May 2020. https://aibolita.com/surgical-treatment/52869-forehead-anatomy.html.
2. Forehead Anatomy: Surface Anatomy, Bones of the Forehead, Forehead and Scalp, 19 February 2020. https://emedicine.medscape.com/article/834862-overview?pa=9MvXuFaoPmIwI3Rk4%2B%2FgI678O DTn10E3dqNllX8w%2F0HbORhYYi63zo0V2AImT8YHfNDL%2FblMpKBX7yWW5h%2FjnichrzF %2F7vlnSF6AEX%2F09M8%3D.
3. Rossetto O, Pirazzini M, Fabris F, Montecucco C, "Botulinum neurotoxins: Mechanism of action," *Handbook of Experimental Pharmacology*, 11 April 2020. https://doi.org/–10.1007/164_2020_355.

4

The Periorbital Region

Vincent Wong

CONTENTS

The periorbital region covers the area and structures surrounding the bony margin of the orbital rim. This includes the eyelids, eyebrows, infraorbital regions, and the temples (see Figure 4.1). As signs of chronological and photoageing in these regions jointly contribute to the general appearance of senescence around the eyes, successful non-surgical rejuvenation usually requires a combination of minimally invasive treatments to restore volume, resurface wrinkles, improve pigmentation, and smooth the mimetic muscles of the face.

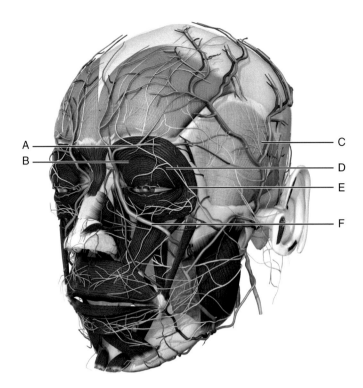

FIGURE 4.1 Structures of the periorbital region: A, supra-orbital vein; B, orbicularis oculi, orbital; C, temporalis; D, orbicularis oculi, palpebral; E, facial nerve, zygomatic branches; F, facial vein. (Adapted from www.anatomy.tv with permission © Informa UK Ltd [trading as Primal Pictures], 2021.)

Tear Trough Deformity and Infraorbital Volume Loss

The tear trough is a hollow that runs along the medial part of the orbital rim, from the medial canthus to the midpupillary line [1, 2]. The area of depression is thought to be secondary to the lack of underlying fat at the insertion of orbicularis oculi muscle inferior to the orbital rim, and the absence of subcutaneous fat [1]. This groove is also enhanced by the medial palpebral bag above and the superficial cheek fat below it [1, 3]. Clinically, patients often present with darkness and hollowing in the tear trough region, giving them a fatigued appearance that is difficult to conceal with makeup products. This darkness is also partially due to thin, pigmented skin covering the area and the absence of subcutaneous fat, which allows the dark colour of the muscle to show. Sadick et al proposed that tear trough deformity is often related to the projection of the upper cheek and that it may be more common in patients with either congenital or age-related maxillary hypoplasia [2]. When the cheek bone is relatively posterior to the projection of the eyeball or the front of the cornea, a negative vector is created which can contribute to the appearance of eye circles (Figure 4.2).

Atrophy of the subcutaneous fat under the eyes is commonly observed with age [3]. When mild and confined to the orbital rim, it gives rise to the palpebromalar groove by exposing the angle between the orbital septum and orbital rim [1]. With the ageing process, this atrophy becomes more extensive and gives the impression of a longer lower eyelid with a lower lid-cheek junction (Figure 4.3).

In a youthful face, the transition between the pre-septal portion (overlying the orbital septum) and orbital portions of the orbicular oculi muscle should be smooth, and this should be continuous with the upper malar region without a transition point. It is important to note that dark circles around the eyes

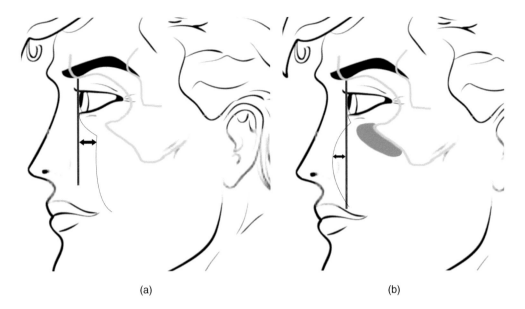

(a)   (b)

FIGURE 4.2 Relationship between tear trough deformity and the projection of the upper cheek. (a) A negative vector, where the eyes are more forward compared to the cheeks, can contribute to the appearance of under eye circles. (b) This can be corrected with dermal fillers to bring the cheeks and malar fat pad forward.

are often multi-factorial. Apart from volume loss, changes in skin thickness, laxity, hyperpigmentation, actinic changes, and prominent subcutaneous venous pooling also play a role.

Severity Assessment

It is important to rate the severity of infraorbital volume loss before starting treatment. The scale in Figure 4.4 acts as a tool to help in the clinical assessment of the patient.

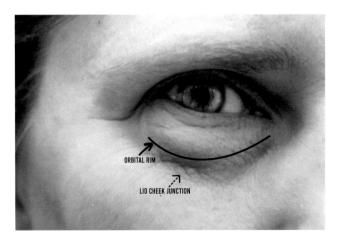

FIGURE 4.3 Extensive atrophy of subcutaneous fat gives the impression of a longer lower eyelid with a lower lid-cheek junction.

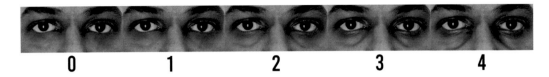

0   1   2   3   4

FIGURE 4.4   Infraorbital hollowness severity scale. 0 = no hollowness, 1 = mild hollowness, 2 = moderate hollowness, 3 = severe hollowness, 4 = very severe hollowness.

Treatment Options

Dermal Fillers

Good patient satisfaction has been observed with hyaluronic acid (HA) dermal fillers treatment with differing degradation profiles [4, 5]. The ideal HA dermal filler for this anatomical region should be:

a. Cross-linked to ensure longevity of the treatment
b. Weakly hydrophilic and made up of small-sized HA particles to avoid extensive oedema and fluid retention
c. Combined with lidocaine, for extra patient comfort

A variety of techniques have evolved over the years to address the tear trough and infraorbital region. Needles and cannulas are widely used by physicians, and there are safety data in the literature to support the use of both [4–6].

25G and 28G cannulas can be used to treat the infraorbital region. Cannulas are usually introduced into the deep fat layer 1.5 cm below the temporal orbital rim. The cannula should progress naturally into the fat under the orbicularis oculi muscle – injections should be slow and gentle; on average, 0.5–0.8 ml of HA filler is required on either side.

Only superficial injections are required when correcting the palpebromalar groove as the etiology is atrophy of superficial fat. 28G cannula can be used for this treatment, introduced just below the lateral canthus and progressed along the palpebromalar groove.

Autologous Cell Therapy (Fat and Platelet)

The use of patient's own cells to enhance aesthetic appearance has long been a practice in medicine. Autologous fat transfer is a classic example of such practice, where fat cells are harvested from a donor site, processed, and then transferred to a recipient site. For facial rejuvenation, harvested fat cells can be used in the same way as dermal fillers. As the cells are taken from the patient, there is no risk of allergic or hypersensitivity reactions, and the risk of encapsulation and granuloma formation (as sometimes observed with some dermal fillers) is eliminated. Traditionally, fat harvesting was done through surgical liposuction. However, development in technology and scientific research has led to a safer, non-surgical method of harvesting fat using microcannula, which can be performed in a sterile clinical room.

In the last decade, there has also been a huge rise in the use of autologous platelets (both platelet-rich and platelet-poor plasma) for facial rejuvenation. The high concentrations of a range of growth factors are thought to help repair and restore the injected area to a younger state, through angiogenesis, neocollagenesis, and thickening of the skin [7]. Platelet-containing plasma is injected directly into the infraorbital area through a series of deep and superficial injections.

Recent studies have also shown that combining autologous platelets and fat cells can enhance the outcome and longevity of autologous treatments. The growth factors from the platelets are thought to improve the survival rate of the fat cells by increasing the proliferation and differentiation of adipose-derived stem cells (ASCs) into adipocytes, improve fat graft vascularisation, and may block the apoptosis of grafted adipocytes [8, 9]. The combination may also improve the cutaneous trophicity above the grafted areas [8]. As the grafted fat is not as viscous or volumising as HA gels, the volume injected is usually higher, starting from an average of 2 ml per side [8].

Combination of Treatments

- Skin peel (mid-depth)
- Mesotherapy (e.g. HA and vitamins)
- Laser resurfacing (e.g. YAG or IPL)
- Growth factor induced therapy

Complications

- Haematoma (needle trauma)
- Retrograde embolism (usually with a needle)
- Vessel and nerve compression (from overfilling or using a hydrophilic filler)
- Lymphatic statis (from damage to lymphatic system)
- Irregular edges (incorrect product placement or migration)
- Oedema (needle trauma or hydrophilic filler)
- Infection (lack of aseptic technique)
- Granuloma formation (reaction to dermal filler)
- Tyndall effect (superficial injections)
- Diplopia (occlusion or compression of neurovascular bundle)
- Necrosis and/or blindness (occlusion of vessel)
- Donor and recipient site unevenness (from fat harvest and fat apoptosis) [8, 9].

Crow's Feet

Crow's feet are rhytides around the lateral canthus. These wrinkles usually develop as a result of increased muscle tone of the orbicularis oculi. As the muscle is firmly attached to the overlying skin, crow's feet usually develop perpendicular to the direction of the muscle fibres.

The severity of crow's feet can be assessed using the following scale (Figure 4.5), which allows the practitioner to assess both dynamic and static rhytides.

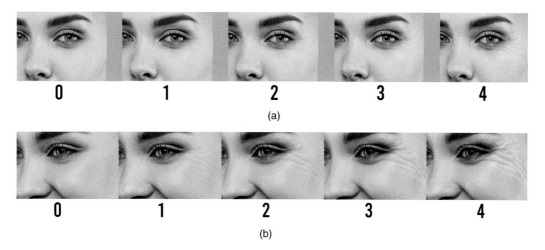

FIGURE 4.5   (a) Crow's feet severity scale (at rest). (b) Crow's feet severity scale (on animation). 0 = no wrinkle, 1 = mild wrinkles, 2 = moderate wrinkles, 3 = severe wrinkles, 4 = very severe wrinkles (following the scales of Merz Aesthetics).

Treatment Options

Neuromodulator (Botulinum Toxin Type A)

Botulinum toxin type A therapy is very popular among physicians and patients as it is safe, simple, effective, and predictable. The musculature and muscle movements in the periorbital area are particularly well suited for neuromodulator treatments. Indeed, the crow's feet region is one of the most popular sites to benefit from the aesthetic result of type A toxin application. The aim of the treatment is to soften the appearance of dynamic and static lines that are caused by the muscle tone of the underlying orbicularis oculi muscle [10]. It is important to note that the goal of neuromodulator injection in this region should be muscle weakening, not paralysis, as natural expressions and movements should still be maintained for a more pleasing outcome. On average three injections of 2.5 standard units of botulinum toxin type A are required around each lateral canthus (in a C shape). The smoother, line-free skin from this treatment typically lasts for 3–4 months; however, repeated treatments have been shown to improve its longevity [10, 11].

Polydioxanone Threads

Polydioxanone (PDO) is a crystalline, biodegradable synthetic non-animal-based polymer that is colourless [12]. It is chemically based on a polymeric structure composed of multiple repeating units of ether-ester and is obtained by ring-opening polymerisation of the monomer p-dioxanone. With a long safety record in surgery, PDO threads are hydrolysed over 6–8 months and eliminated via the kidneys [12, 13]. The aim of treatment using PDO threads in the periorbital region is wrinkle and skin quality improvement. Hence, monofilament PDO threads are often used in this region. Multi-monofilament-PDO scaffolds in the skin have been shown to be safe and effective in reducing the appearance of wrinkles; increased density of threads (by placing them closer together or in multiple layers) creates a denser structural framework for tissue support [12]. The monofilaments induce collagenesis via foreign body reaction which promotes tissue contraction through wound healing. In addition, elastic fibrosis around the treated area has also been observed and contributes towards the aesthetics outcome [12]. Monofilament PDO threads are usually placed in the dermis; horizontally and obliquely around the lateral canthus, with further threads inserted perpendicular to the direction of these threads. The number of monofilament threads used for this region varies between patients – on average 15–30 threads are inserted per side. In Asia, the number of threads used is much higher, in the region of 50 threads and above per side.

Combination of Treatments

- PDO (monofilament threads) combined with neuromodulator
- Laser resurfacing treatments (e.g. YAG and IPL)
- Mesotherapy (e.g. DMAE, HA and vitamins)
- Growth factor induced therapy
- Temple enhancement with dermal fillers (highly cohesive HA)
- Eyebrow lift

Complications

- Swelling (from needle trauma)
- Bruising (from needle trauma)
- Infection (lack of aseptic technique)
- Formation or worsening of malar mounds and/or festoons (due to weakening of the orbicularis oculi muscle)

Temple Hollowness

The temple region is defined by the following boundaries [1]:

- Superiorly by the temporal crest
- Anteriorly by the external orbital rim
- Inferiorly by the zygomatic arch
- Posteriorly by the posterior portion of the superior temporal line (a landmark for this would be the top of the mastoid process)

Volume loss in the temple is one of the earliest but often unaddressed signs of facial ageing. Hollowness and concavity in the temple region, as a result of fat and muscle volume loss, contribute to the appearance of droopy lateral eyebrows and eyelids, and can also create the appearance of exposed zygoma in thin patients. As a result, patients with deep hollows in this region usually appear tired and undernourished, with distorted facial harmony and balance.

Severity Assessment

The scale in Figure 4.6 acts as a tool to help in the clinical assessment of the severity of temple hollowness.

Treatment Options

Dermal Fillers

The most effective treatment to revolumise this area would be the strategic placement of dermal fillers. Treatment of this region usually produces satisfying results. There are two different injection techniques; deep and superficial [1].

Deep injections are performed with a long 27G needle. The aim is to deposit the filler on the periosteum. The superior medial quadrant of the temple is generally regarded as a safe zone for supraperiosteal placement of dermal fillers. The needle is usually introduced perpendicular to the skin surface and advanced until it makes contact with the bone. The entry point is the point of deepest depression in the superior medial quadrant (usually 1 cm above the orbital rim and 1 cm lateral to the temporal crest), and highly cohesive HA filler is injected slowly. Usually 2–3 ml of product is required per side.

21–25G cannulas are usually used for superficial injections with a moderately cohesive HA filer. Two to three openings with an introducer needle are usually required; typical locations include lateral canthus, middle third of the eyebrow and at the hairline above the root of Helix [1]. Fillers are placed in the loose areolar tissue in between the temporoparietal fascia and the deep temporal fascia (Figure 4.7). On average, 1–2 ml of product is injected per side.

Autologous Fat Transfer

Fat cells harvested from the patient and enriched with PRP to enhance the survival rate of adipocytes can be injected in this anatomical region, both superficially and through deep, supraperiosteal injections [8, 9].

  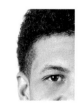 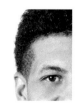 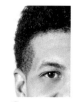

0 - Convex 1 - Flat 2 - Minimal 3 - Moderate 4 - Severe

FIGURE 4.6 Temple hollowness severity scale. 0 = convex, 1 = flat, 2 = minimal hollowness, 3 = moderate hollowness, 4 = severe hollowness.

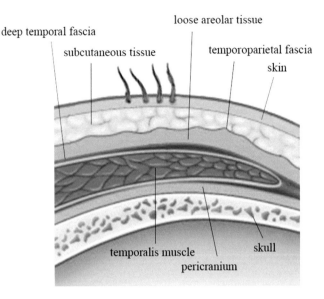

FIGURE 4.7   Cross section of the temple region.

The abundance of adipose tissue means that higher volumes can be used for facial rejuvenation. Many patients who had autologous fat injected in the temple and forehead region also noticed significant change to their eyebrow position, and this is likely due to the volume injected (average 5.9 ml per temple) [14, 15].

Combination Treatments

- Eyebrow lift
- Crow's feet treatments
- Mesotherapy (e.g. vitamins and HA)
- Skin peel (superficial or mid-depth)
- Laser skin resurfacing (e.g. YAG or IPL)
- Growth factor induced therapy

Complications

- Blindness (due to the multitude of vessels that course through this region at various depth) [16, 17]
- Swelling (from needle trauma)
- Bruising (from needle trauma)
- Infection (lack of aseptic technique)
- Lumpiness (incorrect product placement or migration)
- Ptosis (compression of neurovascular bundle)
- Ophthalmoplegia (compression of neurovascular bundle)
- Granuloma formation (reaction to dermal filler)

Eyelid Hooding

The eyelids are the protective covering of the ocular globe. The skin of the eyelid is the thinnest on the human body. The upper eyelid extends superiorly and is separated from the forehead by the eyebrow [18]. The lower eyelid extends below the inferior orbital border and is juxtaposed to the thicker tissue of the

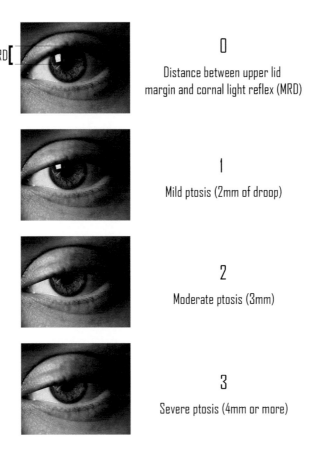

FIGURE 4.8 Marginal reflex distance. 0 = no ptosis (MRD = 4 mm), 1 = mild ptosis of 2 mm (MRD = 2 mm), 2 = moderate ptosis of 3 mm (MRD = 1 mm), 3 = severe ptosis of 4 mm or more (MRD less than 1 mm).

cheek [1, 18]. The palpebral borders of the upper and lower eyelids come in contact during the closure and the blinking movement of the eyelids. Apart from protecting the globe, the eyelids also help in creating and maintaining the lacrimal film, which is necessary for corneal survival.

A decrease in the distance of the palpebral fissure is quite common with ageing and typically presents with palpebral ptosis (lowering of the upper eyelid) and/or dermatochalasis (excessive skin of the eyelids). The degree of eyelid hooding can be categorised by measuring the marginal reflex distance (Figure 4.8). From the point where light is reflected from the pupil, the distance to the upper eyelid should be between 4 and 4.5 mm. Anything less indicates a heavy or droopy upper eyelid.

Treatment Options

Plasma Ionisation

Plasma ionisation (PI) is a relative new addition to the aesthetics field and has gained high popularity in recent years. PI works through the non-ablative process of sublimation. Plasma (fourth state of matter) is formed through the ionisation of atmospheric gas, which works to stimulate the contraction, shortening, and tightening of skin fibres, thus resulting in the reduction of the skin surface. For periorbital rejuvenation, PI has been highly effective in tightening the skin around the upper and lower eyelids, offering patients an alternative to surgical blepharoplasty, reducing recovery time and any complications that can arise before and after surgery [19]. The advantages of using PI include instant results and no damage to surrounding tissues as no heat is transferred to the surrounding area. The resultant tissue retraction and tightening (as opposed to removal) gives results that are comparable to the ones seen with invasive surgery [19]. As with all non-surgical treatments, patient selection is an important factor. This treatment works best in mild to moderate cases of excessive or loose skin in the upper eyelids. The upper eyelid is treated in a dot-to-dot approach. Each dot is a treatment point and is located approximately 2 mm away from the next. The end point of treatment is the formation of a brown crust on each dot. On average, treatment takes approximately 15 minutes per side.

Dermal Fillers

HA fillers are injected in the supratarsal fold in patients with volume loss in the area leading to ptosis of the upper eyelid [1]. The use of a 25 or 27G cannula is advisable, with an entry point lateral to the mid-pupillary line to avoid the supraorbital neurovascular bundle. Filler is placed in the periosteal plane, following the orbital rim. Care must be taken to avoid injection below the orbital rim. Placing a finger (of the non-injecting hand) just under the orbital rim during injections provides support to the tissue and protection to the globe. On average, 0.2–0.4 ml of dermal fillers is injected per side.

Combination of Treatments

- Crow's feet treatment (e.g. neuromodulator)
- Eyebrow lift
- Temple filling with highly cohesive dermal fillers
- Mesotherapy to surrounding area (e.g. vitamins, HA)

Complications

- Globe involvement (incorrect placement of needle/cannula/product)
- Extensive oedema (needle trauma)
- Extensive bruising (supratrochlear and supraorbital neurovascular bundles)
- Crusting and scabbing (PI treatment)
- Infection (lack of aseptic technique)
- Pigmentation (lack of protection against sun damage)

Eyebrow Position

The eyebrows frame the eyes and are a prominent feature of the face. They are composed of five layers as follow [1]:

1. Skin (dense sebaceous and sweat glands as well as hair follicles)
2. Loose connective tissue with multiple structures crossing to connect to the overlying skin from the underlying muscular layer
3. Muscle tissue
4. Loose cellular tissue
5. Periosteum

The muscle layer can be further divided into superficial layer (frontalis and orbicularis oculi) and deep layer (corrugator). These two layers often intertwine at different heights in the eyebrow, accounting for the muscular balance and hence eyebrow position [1].

The 4th layer (loose cellular tissue) is continuous with the frontal space under the galea. This is where the eyebrow commonly slides with age. Figure 4.9 shows the eyebrow droopiness severity scale, which can be used as a tool for clinical assessment.

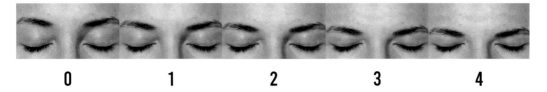

FIGURE 4.9 Eyebrow droopiness severity scale. 0 = no droop, 1 = mild droop, 2 = moderate droop, 3 = severe droop, 4 = very severe droop (following the scale of Merz Aesthetics).

Treatment Options

Neuromodulator (Botulinum Toxin Type A)

The frontalis muscle works to raise the eyebrows, whereas the orbicularis oculi and corrugator work to pull the eyebrows down and in an inferomedial direction. Hence, an eyebrow lift can be achieved by strategically weakening the corrugator and the orbicularis oculi muscles. This would allow the frontalis muscle to work unopposed. In general, one injection of 2.5 standard units of botulinum toxin type A at the lateral end of the eyebrow and two 5-standard-unit injections in the corrugator (in the medial and lateral portions) per side are sufficient to achieve a noticeable lift. However, it is also important to note that an eyebrow droop could be the result of overdose of botulinum toxin type A in the frontalis – in which case, it is best to let the effects of the toxin wear off naturally.

Filler

For this anatomical region, 25–27G cannulas are recommended for the injection of moderately cross-linked dermal filler. The eyebrows are highly vascular, as branches from the supratrochlear, supra-orbital, superficial temporal, and lacrimal arteries cross and form anastomoses at various layers to emerge above the muscles in the forehead [1]. Additionally, there is an extensive venous network draining towards the medial canthus. Lateral and medial injection techniques can be used when treating the eyebrow, with insertion points under the lateral end of the eyebrow and lateral to the midpupillary line above the eyebrow respectively [1]. Regardless of the technique, it is important to ensure that the cannula is inserted on top of the orbital rim and that the filler is injected supraperiosteally. The filler (0.2–0.4 ml on average) must also be deposited at the superior margin of the eyebrow and slightly below it to create an ascending effect [1].

Threads

As the eyebrows slide with age, a wide range of resorbable threads can be inserted into the subcutaneous layer of the forehead to lift the eyebrows. The common materials include PDO, polylactic acid, and polycaprolactone. Apart from stimulating collagen production and achieving an overall tightening effect on the skin, these threads also help to reposition soft tissue with the barbs and cones on them [12, 13]. The soft tissue and overlying skin are mechanically lifted by attaching the threads to specific anchoring points. The number of threads ranges from 1 to 5, depending on the type of thread and their lifting capacity.

Combination of Treatments

- Combination of neuromodulator, threads, and filler
- Eyelid treatments (e.g. PI and neuromodulator)
- Temple volumisation with highly cohesive dermal fillers

Complications

- Eyebrow droop (incorrect dosage or placement of neuromodulator)
- Venous compression and/or necrosis (incorrect placement of dermal fillers)
- Extensive swelling (needle trauma)
- Extensive bruising (needle trauma)
- Skin puckering (from thread treatments, some cases may require mechanical release with a needle)
- Fibrosis (from thread treatments)
- Infection (lack of aseptic technique)

Case Study 4.1

Patient Age: 49
   Sex: Female
   Presenting Concern: Crow's feet
   Grading (before): 3 (severe) (Figure 4.10)

Treatment Plan

- Botulinum toxin using Botox by Allergan (7.5 units to each side of the periorbital region, 15 units in total) (Figure 4.11)

Grading (after): 0 (none)

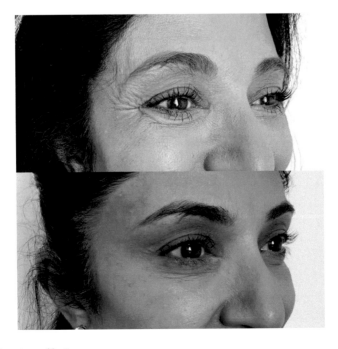

FIGURE 4.10   Patient: top and bottom.

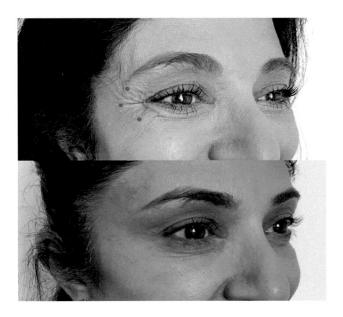

FIGURE 4.11   Blue dots, 2.5 u Botox per injection.

Case Study 4.2

Patient Age: 38
  Sex: Male
  Presenting Concern: Tear trough and infraorbital hollow (palpebromalar groove)
  Grading (before): 3 (severe) (Figure 4.12)

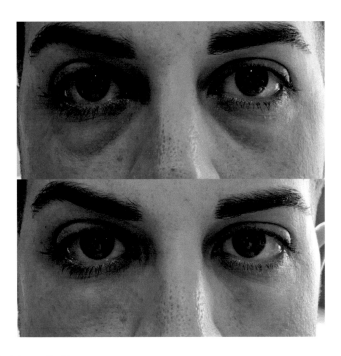

FIGURE 4.12   Patient: top and bottom.

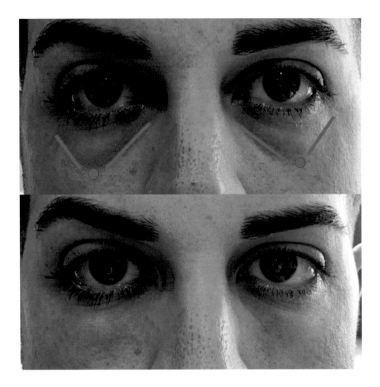

FIGURE 4.13   Straight line: retrograde linear technique; circle, bolus technique.

Treatment Plan

- *Session 1*: Dermal filler using Definisse Restore by Relife (1 ml per side, 2 ml in total) (Figure 4.13)
- *Session 2*: Mesotherapy using NCTF-135HA by FillMed (Figure 4.14)

Grading (after): 0 (none)

Case Study 4.3

Patient Age: 40
 Sex: Female
 Presenting Concern: Increased skin laxity of upper and lower eyelids, minimal upper eyelid hooding and infraorbital wrinkles (Figure 4.15)

Treatment Plan

- PI using Jett Plasma (1 session) (Figures 4.16 and 4.17)

Outcome

Tightening of upper and lower eyelids, infraorbital region as well as reduction in infraorbital wrinkles.

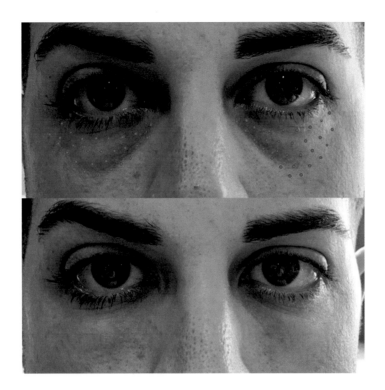

FIGURE 4.14 Blue dots, serial puncture technique.

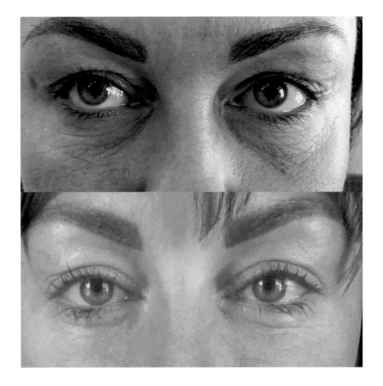

FIGURE 4.15 Patient: top and bottom.

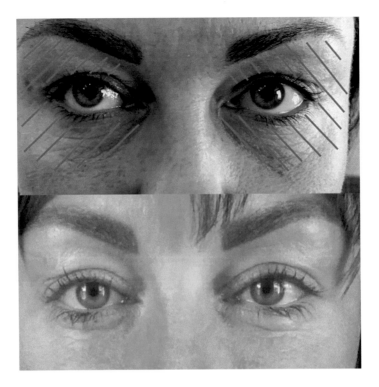

FIGURE 4.16   Straight lines, scanning technique.

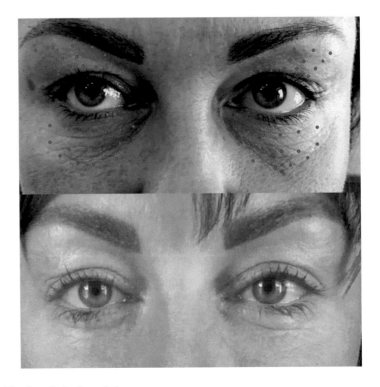

FIGURE 4.17   Blue dots, dot by dot technique.

REFERENCES

1. Andre P, Garcia P. *Anatomy and Volumising Injections*. UK: E2e Medical Pub; 2012.
2. Sadick N, Bosniak S, Cantisano-Zilkha M, Glavas I, Roy D, "Definition of the tear trough and the tear trough rating scale," *Journal of Cosmetic Dermatology*, vol. 6, no. 4, pp. 218–222, 2007.
3. Gierloff M, Stohring C, Buder T, Wiltfang J, "The subcutaneous fat compartments in relation to aesthetically important facial folds and rhytides," *Journal of Plastic, Reconstructive & Aesthetic Surgery*, vol. 65, no. 10, pp. 1292–1297, 2012.
4. De Pasquale A, Russa G, Pulvirenti M, Di Rosa L, "Hyaluronic acid filler injections for tear-trough deformity: Injection technique and high-frequency ultrasound follow-up evaluation," *Aesthetic Plastic Surgery*, vol. 37, no. 3, pp. 587–591, 2013.
5. Sattler G, "The tower technique and vertical supraperiosteal depot technique: Novel vertical injection techniques for volume-efficient subcutaneous tissue support and volumetric augmentation," *Journal of Drugs in Dermatology*, vol. 11, no. 8, pp. s45-s47, 2012.
6. Berros P, Lax L, Bétis F, "Hyalurostructure treatment," *Plastic and Reconstructive Surgery*, vol. 132, no. 6, pp. 924e–931e.
7. Cameli N, Mariano M, Cordone I, Abril E, Masi S, Foddai M, "Autologous pure platelet-rich plasma dermal injections for facial skin rejuvenation," *Dermatologic Surgery*, vol. 43, no. 6, pp. 826–835, 2017.
8. Picard F, Hersant B, La Padula S, Meningaud J, "Platelet-rich plasma-enriched autologous fat graft in regenerative and aesthetic facial surgery: Technical note," *Journal of Stomatology, Oral and Maxillofacial Surgery*, 2017. Available at: http://dx.doi.org/10.1016/j.jormas.2017.05.005 [Accessed 4 Sep. 2017].
9. James I, Coleman S, Rubin J, "Fat, stem cells, and platelet-rich plasma," *Clinics in Plastic Surgery*, vol. 43, no. 3, pp. 473–488, 2016.
10. Gendler E, Nagler A, "Aesthetic use of BoNT: Options and outcomes," *Toxicon*, vol. 107, pp. 120–128, 2015.
11. Carruthers A, Bruce S, de Coninck A, et al. "Efficacy and safety of onabotulinumtoxinA for the treatment of crows feet lines," *Dermatologic Surgery*, vol. 40, no. 11, pp. 1181–1190, 2014.
12. Kim H, Bae I, Ko H, Choi J, Park Y, Park W, "Novel polydioxanone multifilament scaffold device for tissue regeneration," *Dermatologic Surgery*, vol. 42, no. 1, pp. 63–67, 2016.
13. De Masi F, De Masi R, De Masi E, "Suspension threads," *Facial Plastic Surgery*, vol. 32, no. 06, pp. 662–663, 2016.
14. Chiu C, "Objective evaluation of eyebrow position after autologous fat grafting to the temple and forehead," *Aesthetic Plastic Surgery*, 2017. Available at: http://dx.doi.org/10.1007/s00266-017-0881-4 [Accessed 4 Sep. 2017].
15. Shue S, Kurlander D, Guyuron B, Fat injection: A systematic review of injection volumes by facial subunit. *Aesthetic Plastic Surgery*, 2017. Available at: http://dx.doi.org/10.1007/s00266-017-0936-6 [Accessed 4 Sep. 2017].
16. Chen Y, "Fundus artery occlusion caused by cosmetic facial injections," *Chinese Medical Journal (Engl)*, vol. 127, no. 8, pp. 1434–1437, 2014.
17. Breithaupt A, Jones D, Braz A, Narins R, Weinkle S, "Anatomical basis for safe and effective volumization of the temple," *Dermatologic Surgery*, vol. 41, pp. S278–S283, 2015.
18. Goldberg R. "Eyelid anatomy revisited," *Archives of Ophthalmology*, vol. 110, no. 11, pp. 1598, 1992.
19. Rossi E. "Applications of plasma exeresis in dermatology," *Aesthetic Medicine*, vol. 32, no. 11, pp. e411–e413, 2016.

5

The Nose

Vincent Wong

CONTENTS

The nose is arguably the most prominent feature of the face. It is made up of a fixed part (formed by the frontal notch, parts of the zygomatic and nasal bones, the upper lateral cartilage, and the septum) and a mobile part (formed by the lower lateral cartilage and the lower part of the upper lateral cartilage) [1]. See further in Figure 5.1.

When planning aesthetic enhancement procedures, we must consider the nose as a stand-alone unit with its specific volumes as well as a part of the face with specific ratios that have to be respected to achieve overall facial harmony. The two key angles that are crucial in achieving this harmony are:

1. *Naso-frontal angle*: This is assessed on profile view and reflects the angle between the glabella and the dorsum of the nose. Ideally, this should be 115–135 degrees, with 130 degrees being the ideal for men and 135 degrees being the ideal for women (Figure 5.1) [2, 3].

2. *Nasolabial angle*: This angle, also assessed on profile view, is formed between the columella and the upper lip. This should be between 90–95 degrees in men and 95–100 degrees in women (Figure 5.2) [2, 3].

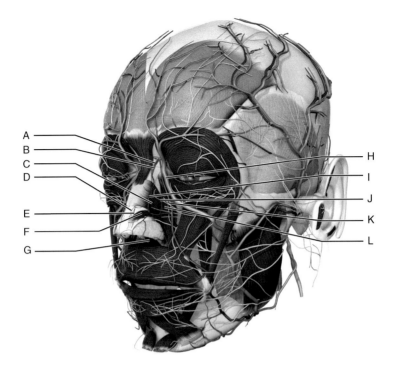

FIGURE 5.1   Structures of the nose: A, dorsal nasal vein; B, dorsal nasal artery; C, nasalis, transverse part (compressor); D, anterior ethmoid vein; E, anterior ethmoid artery; F, nasalis, alar part; dilator); G, depressor septi (depressor); H, facial vein; I, lateral nasal artery; J, facial nerve, zygomatic branches; K, facial artery; L, levator labii superioris alaeque nasi (levator). (Adapted from www.anatomy.tv with permission © Informa UK Ltd [trading as Primal Pictures], 2021.)

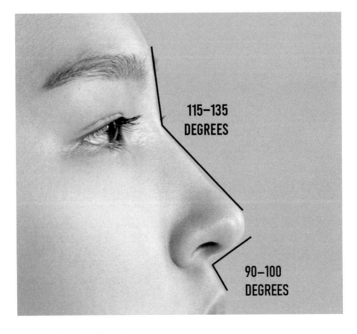

FIGURE 5.2   Naso-frontal and nasolabial angles.

In addition, enhancement of the lips and chin with dermal fillers can also help us achieve overall facial harmony. In certain cases, the nose may appear smaller or less protruding when balanced correctly with chin and lips enhancements (medical profiloplasty).

The layers of the nose, from superficial to deep, include [4]:

1. *Skin*: The skin is thin at the nose bridge and gets progressively thicker towards the tip. In the mobile part, the skin also has more dense sebaceous glands.
2. *Cellular subcutaneous tissue*: This layer is relatively underdeveloped and forms a clear layer with very little fat in the mobile part of the nose.
3. *Muscles*: This layer contains elevator, depressor, compressor, and dilator muscles for the nostrils.
4. *Perichondro-periosteal envelope*: This layer is made up of interconnected fibres and holds together the structures of the nasal pyramid.
5. *Vessels and nerves*: Vessels are generally small and located at the sides of the nose. Motor branches of the facial nerve are interconnected through the nasal superficial musculoaponeurotic system to supply the muscles.

Naso-Frontal Angle and Dorsal Hump

The correction of naso-frontal angle and dorsal hump are the most common requests for non-surgical nose enhancement. These issues are more prominent in certain ethnic groups: for example, many Chinese patients have a very low nasal bridge and hence would seek correction of the naso-frontal angle to achieve harmony between facial features.

Severity Assessment

The ideal naso-frontal angle is between 115 and 135 degrees (as mentioned above). To assess the clinical severity of a dorsal hump, the scale in Figure 5.3 acts as a tool to help in patient evaluation.

Treatment Option

Dermal Filler

Different volumising fillers have been used in medical rhinoplasties. Apart from having a high safety profile, the injected product must also have the ability to diffuse in the filled spaces. Hence, non-resorbable products are not recommended for this anatomical region, and hyaluronic acid fillers remain the product of choice.

To correct or enhance the naso-frontal angle, a highly cross-linked hyaluronic acid should be used with a 27G needle. Injections should only be made in the midline to avoid blood vessels. The needle should be introduced at an angle of 45 degrees until it reaches the periosteum. The thumb and index finger of the non-dominant hand

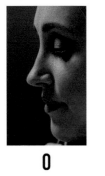 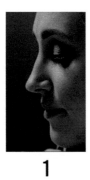 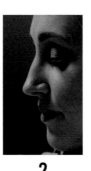 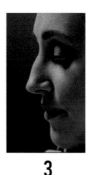 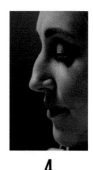

0   **1**   **2**   **3**   **4**

FIGURE 5.3 Dorsal hump severity scale. 0 = no dorsal hump, 1 = mild dorsal hump, 2 = moderate dorsal hump, 3 = severe dorsal hump, 4 = very severe dorsal hump.

should exert pressure on the lateral walls of the nasal bone to prevent spreading of the filler into the lower eyelid and tear trough. Usually, 0.2–0.3 ml is sufficient to achieve aesthetically pleasing results.

For dorsal humps, hyaluronic acid filler with high cross-linking should be injected superior and inferior to the bump to achieve a smooth contour of the nose. For safety reasons, injections should be made along the midline. Generally, more volume will be required superior to the dorsal hump, but 0.3–0.4 ml in total should be sufficient.

Combination of Treatments

- Neuromodulator (botulinum toxin type A)
- Skin peel (superficial)
- Chin and lips enhancement with dermal fillers

Complications

- Haematoma (needle trauma)
- Necrosis (vessel occlusion or compression)
- Under eye oedema (spreading of product)
- Irregular edges (incorrect product placement)
- Oedema (needle trauma or hydrophilic filler)
- Infection (lack of aseptic technique)
- Tyndall effect (superficial injections)

Bunny Lines

Bunny lines are wrinkles that form across the ridge of the nose and the lateral aspects of the nose. They are usually more prominent with facial expressions, such as frowning. As with all dynamic lines, bunny lines tend to get progressively deeper with age due to development of muscle tone (nasalis muscle) and age-related changes to the skin. Some patients may notice the development of bunny lines after neuromodulator treatment to the glabella and forehead – this is due to increased use of the nose in facial expressions secondary to immobilisation of other facial mimetic muscles.

Severity Assessment

The scale in Figure 5.4 acts as a tool to help assess the clinical severity of bunny lines.

Treatment Option

Neuromodulator (Botulinum Toxin Type A)

Bunny lines are commonly treated with a neuromodulator with excellent results. At the point of maximum nasalis contraction at the side of the nose, 4–5 units of botulinum toxin type A can be injected to

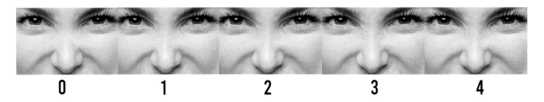

FIGURE 5.4   Bunny line severity scale (on animation). 0 = no wrinkle, 1 = mild wrinkles, 2 = moderate wrinkles, 3 = severe wrinkles, 4 = very severe wrinkles (following the scale of Merz Aesthetics).

relax the muscle. As with all neuromodulator treatments, it can take up to 2 weeks to achieve the optimum result from one treatment. In order to avoid injecting the surrounding muscles, injections are made away from the nose-cheek junction.

Combination of Treatments

- Skin peel (superficial)
- Nose bridge enhancement with dermal fillers

Complications

- Haematoma (needle trauma)
- Drooping of upper lip (injection into surrounding muscles)
- Swelling (needle trauma)
- Infection (lack of aseptic technique)

Nose Tip

Nose tip enhancement is a popular request for both surgical and non-surgical rhinoplasties. Due to its high safety profile, hyaluronic acid can be injected both in the mobile and fixed part of the nose. As a result, subtle but satisfactory changes can be made to the tip of the nose to enhance its shape or to increase its projection and rotation. It is important to manage the patient's expectations accordingly, as medical rhinoplasties can achieve remarkable results in terms of enhancement and camouflage, but they will not dramatically change the size or shape of the nose – which surgical procedures can achieve.

Severity Assessment

Nose projection and rotation can be assessed using the scales in Figures 5.5 and 5.6.

Treatment Options

Dermal Fillers

A highly cross-linked hyaluronic acid dermal filler should be used to ensure a stable outcome. The nose tip is a sensitive area with thicker skin firmly attached to the subcutaneous cartilaginous tissue. As a result, the skin tension is high and injected product tends to extrude if there are too many injection points. Hence, it is recommended that only one or two entry points are created with a 27G needle to distribute the filler in a radial pattern at the tip. On average, 0.2.3 ml of dermal filler is injected slowly and

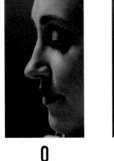 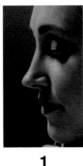 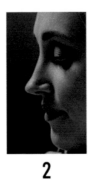 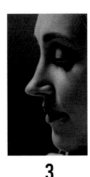 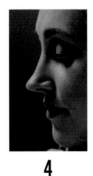

0　　　　**1**　　　　**2**　　　　**3**　　　　**4**

FIGURE 5.5　Nose projection scale. 0 = minimally projected nose tip, 1 = mildly projected nose tip, 2 = moderately projected nose tip, 3 = severely projected nose tip, 4 = very severely projected nose tip.

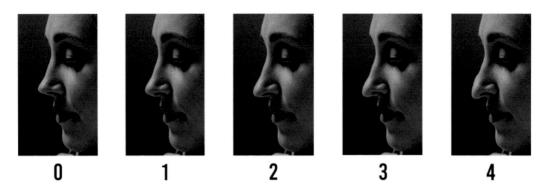

0   1   2   3   4

FIGURE 5.6   Nose tip rotation scale. 0 = severe upward rotation, 1 = mild upward rotation, 2 = horizontal, 3 = mild downward rotation, 4 = severe downward rotation.

steadily to minimise damage or occlusion to the blood vessels which could lead to necrosis. It is important to note that the nose tip should not turn pale as a result of filling (a sign of vascular occlusion). The end result may also be further enhanced with 0.2 ml of the same dermal filler injected supraperiosteally in each alar base. The nose tip will appear softer, narrower, and more defined.

To improve nose tip rotation and/or columellar show, hyaluronic acid dermal filler with high cross-linking can be injected deeply using a 27G needle directly onto the nasal spine (supraperiosteally) in order to open up the nasolabial angle. More superficial injections can be performed to balance the lines of the columella. Usually, 0.2–0.3 ml is required.

Neuromodulator

In some cases, the tip of the nose may project downward during facial expressions such as smiling and laughing. This is due to contraction of the depressor septi muscle and may worsen the natural drooping of the nose tip that occurs with ageing. This can be treated with two units of botulinum toxin type A injected directly beneath the septum.

Some patients may have wide alae that flare easily. This is due to a hyperkinetic alar nasalis muscle. This can be corrected with injections of 5–10 units of botulinum toxin type A to each side. However, this is only suitable for those who can actively and voluntarily flare their nostrils. In these individuals, the treatment will reduce the frontal diameter of the nostrils, hence achieving a narrower nose tip without interfering with inspiration.

Combination of Treatments

- Chin and lips enhancement with dermal fillers

Complications

- Haematoma (needle trauma)
- Necrosis (vessel occlusion or compression)
- Irregular edges (incorrect product placement)
- Oedema (needle trauma or hydrophilic filler)
- Infection (lack of aseptic technique)
- Tyndall effect (superficial injections)

Case Study 5.1

Patient Age: 47
  Sex: Female

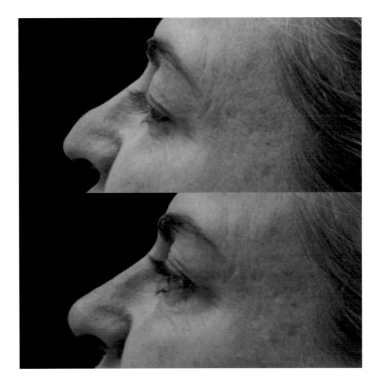

FIGURE 5.7   Patient: top and bottom.

Presenting Concern: Downward nose tip rotation. Patient also seeks improvement of naso-frontal angle.

Grading (before)

- Nose tip rotation: 4 (severe downward rotation)
- Nose tip projection: 0 (minimal) (Figure 5.7)

Treatment Plan

- Dermal filler treatment using Definisse Restore by Relife (1 ml used in total) (Figure 5.8)

Grading (after)

- Nose tip rotation: 2 (horizontal)
- Nose tip projection: 1 (mildly projected)

Case Study 5.2

Patient Age: 25
  Sex: Female
  Presenting Concern: Improvement of nose tip projection
  Grading (before): 0 (minimal) (Figure 5.9)

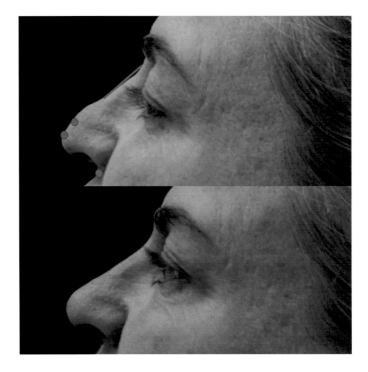

FIGURE 5.8   Straight line, retrograde linear technique; circle, bolus technique.

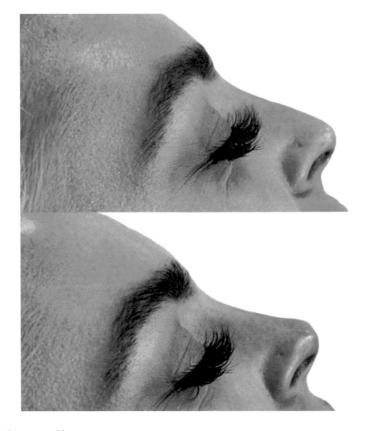

FIGURE 5.9   Patient: top and bottom.

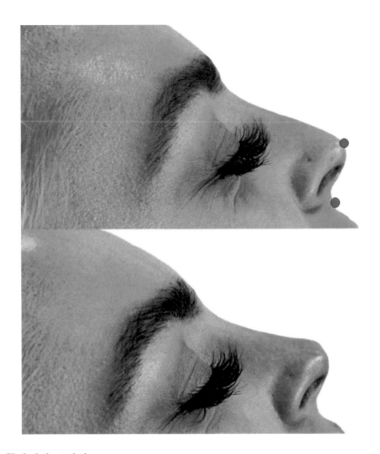

FIGURE 5.10   Circle, bolus technique.

Treatment Plan

- Dermal filler treatment using Definisse Restore by Relife (0.5 ml used in total) (Figure 5.10)

Grading (after): 1 (mildly projected)

REFERENCES

1. Anderson KJ, Henneberg M, Norns RM, "Anatomy of the nasal profile," *Journal of Anatomy*, vol. 213, no. 2, pp. 210–216, 2008.
2. Naini FB, Cobourne MT, Garagiola U, McDonald F, Wertheim D, "Nasofrontal angle and nasal dorsal aesthetics: A quantitative investigation of idealized and normative values," *Facial Plastic Surgery*, vol. 32, no. 4, pp. 444–451, 2016.
3. Ravichandran E, Ravichandran S, "Male vs. female facial rejuvenation," *Aesthetics Journal*, vol. 2, no. 11, 2015.
4. Ozturk CN, Larson JD, Ozturk C, Zins JE, "The SMAS and fat compartments of the nose: An anatomical study," *Aesthetic Plastic Surgery*, vol. 37, no. 1, pp. 11–15, 2013.

6

The Cheeks

Vincent Wong

CONTENTS

Full cheeks are a symbol of youth. Hence, it is no surprise that the cheeks are one of the most treated areas when it comes to facial aesthetics. A full cheek starts at the nasolabial fold and extends to the zygomatic apophysis [1]. With chronological ageing, the loss and redistribution of fat pads, combined with bone changes, lead to a decrease in angularity. As the superficial fat pads are firmly attached to the skin but loosely attached to the superficial muscular aponeurotic system, the loss of volume also leads to pseudoptosis of the skin of the cheek [1]. See Figures 6.1 and 6.2.

Midcheek Groove

The midcheek groove lies in the middle of the cheek, following on from the nasojugal groove – oblique, downwards, and laterally [2]. It defines two distinct anatomical features; the nasolabial fat compartment which lies medial to the midcheek groove and the superficial medial cheek fat compartment which lies lateral to it [2]. See Figure 6.3.

Severity Assessment

The presentation of midcheek groove can range from a mild depression to a median concavity. Severity of midcheek groove correlates with cheek volume. The scale in Figure 6.4 acts as a tool to help in the clinical assessment of the patient.

Treatment Options

- Dermal filler

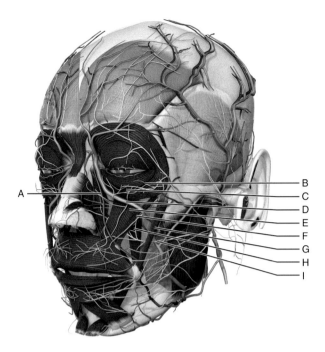

FIGURE 6.1 Structures of the cheeks: A, facial artery; B, facial nerve, zygomatic branches; C, orbicularis oculi, orbital part; D, facial vein; E, levator labii superioris; F, zygomaticus minor; G, zygomaticus major; H, levator labii superioris alaeque nasi; I, facial nerve, upper buccal branches. (Adapted from www.anatomy.tv with permission © Informa UK Ltd [trading as Primal Pictures], 2021.)

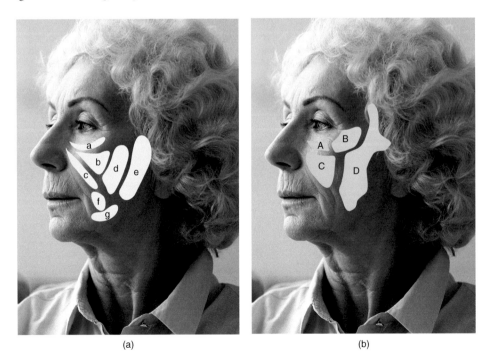

(a)   (b)

FIGURE 6.2   (a) Superficial cheek fat compartments: a, infraorbital fat; b, medial cheek fat; c, nasolabial fat; d, middle cheek fat; e, lateral cheek fat; f, superior jowl fat; g, inferior jowl fat. (b) Deep cheek fat compartments: A, medial sub-orbicularis oculi fat; B, lateral sub-orbicularis oculi fat; C, deep medial cheek fat; D, buccal fat. (Adapted from Fundarò S, Mauro G, Di Blasio A, et al. [2018] Anatomy and aging of cheek fat compartments, *Med Dent* Res. 2: DOI: 10.15761/ MDR.1000111 under Open Access.)

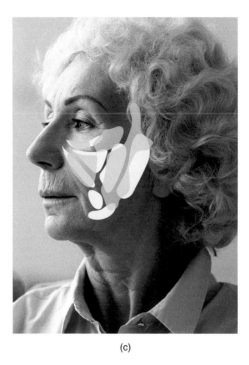

(c)

FIGURE 6.2 (c) Superficial and deep cheek fat compartments in relation to each other. *(Continued)*

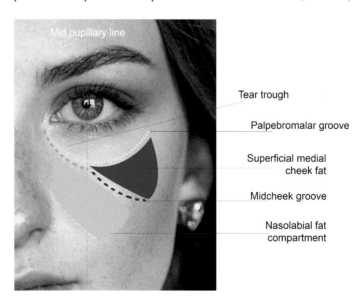

FIGURE 6.3 Location of midcheek groove.

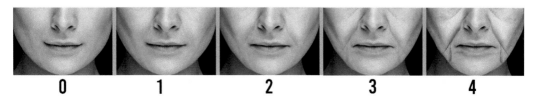

FIGURE 6.4 Midcheek groove severity scale. 0 = full cheeks, 1 = mildly sunken cheeks, 2 = moderately sunken cheeks, 3 = severely sunken cheeks, 4 = very severely sunken cheeks (following the scale of Merz Aesthetics).

As loss of volume is the main cause of midcheek groove, great results can be achieved with volume replacement with dermal fillers. An ideal dermal filler for this region would be:

- Cross-linked to ensure longevity of the treatment. On average, the results from dermal filler placement in this region should last 9–12 months.
- High-viscosity and high-lifting capacity (G′ – elastic modulus) to ensure optimal projection from the injection [3].
- Medium cohesivity to give natural-looking results, with the right balance between tissue integration and stability of the filler [3].
- High G″ (viscous modulus) to ensure precise correction with lower risk of product migration [3].
- Combined with lidocaine for patient comfort.

The patient should be sat up vertically during the procedure to avoid any attenuations from lying down.

The area to be treated should form a triangle lateral to the midcheek groove. Its medial border would be the midcheek groove, lateral side formed by the protuberance of the zygomatic arch, and its upper border the lid-cheek junction [1].

A 25G cannula can be used to effectively refill this area. The dermal filler should be placed supraperiosteally, in a fan shape – starting just laterally to the midcheek groove and progressing to the zygomatic arch (as shown in Figure 6.5) [1].

Deep placement of dermal filler would mean that a greater volume is used during treatment; however, there is a less risk of visible or palpable subcutaneous irregularities with this technique.

In certain patients, more superficial injections would be required. This can be carried out using a second entry point in the zygomatic region [1]. This crossed technique complements corrections in areas where greater volumes have to be restored. See Figure 6.6.

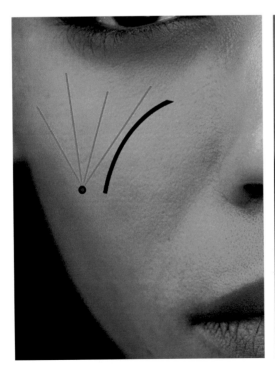 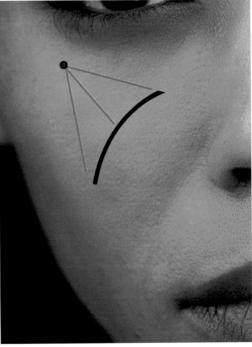

FIGURE 6.5 Deep placement of dermal filler for correction of midcheek groove.

FIGURE 6.6 Superficial placement of dermal filler for midcheek groove correction.

- Bidirectional barbed threads

  The use of facial threads has evolved in recent years and many designs of threads are readily available on the market. The material from which the threads are made of varies from short-lived polydioxanone (PDO) to longer-lasting materials such as polylactic acid and polycaprolactone.

  Bidirectional threads are particularly useful in treating the midcheek groove, as they have the ability to reposition soft tissues in a three-dimensional way, as opposed to the concept of 'lifting', which is two-dimensional. The convergent barbs, when inserted in the superficial fat layer, will hook firmly to the soft tissue – one set of barbs will allow the clinician to effectively reposition the fat pads using a pinching movement (to secure the soft tissue onto the barbs) and by pulling the thread, whilst the other set of barbs acts as anchoring points in the zygoma, where the tissue is less mobile. This technique uses 2–3 threads on each side of the face and is effective in the correction of pseudoptosis of the skin. Longevity of the end result varies according to the thread material and can last up to 24 months with longer lasting materials. See Figure 6.7.

- Autologous fat

  Fat can be harvested from unwanted 'stubborn' areas and reinjected in this region. The concept of revolumisation is similar to dermal filler placement and can be achieved using cannula too. Fat cells treated with platelet-rich plasma have been shown to survive the transfer better, resulting in longer-lasting results [4]. The key differences between dermal fillers and autologous fat are covered in Chapter 11.

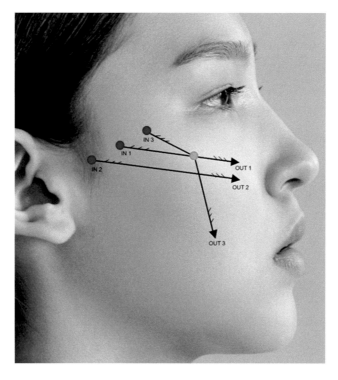

FIGURE 6.7   Positioning of bidirectional convergent threads to reposition soft tissue in the cheeks.

Combination of Treatments

- Dermal filler/fat with threads
- Skin peel
- HIFU
- Mesotherapy
- Laser resurfacing
- Growth factor induced therapy

Complications

- Haematoma
- Skin puckering (from uneven placement of threads)
- Neural pain (from traction of a sensitive nerve branch by threads)
- Vessel and nerve compression (from overfilling or using a hydrophilic filler)
- Lymphatic statis (from damage to lymphatic system)
- Irregular edges
- Oedema
- Infection
- Granuloma formation
- Tyndall effect (superficial injections)
- Necrosis
- Donor and recipient site unevenness (from fat harvest and fat apoptosis)

Cheek Enhancement

The techniques and treatments above can also be used, in the absence of midcheek groove, to enhance the cheek (both medially and laterally). The end result is an improvement in the nasolabial folds, the jawline, and a more contoured midface with enhanced angularity, which may be deemed as attractive by many. If dermal filler is used, it is important to keep the dermal filler placement in the supraperiosteal layer in the zygomatic arch, zygomatic eminence, and anteromedial cheek to prevent any visible irregularities [1]. Filler injections in the submalar and lateral lower cheek (parotid area) should be in the subcutaneous layer [1]. It is also crucial to understand the differences between a male and female face in this region to avoid any unwanted feminisation or masculinisation. MRI studies have shown that the superficial fat layer is 1.5 times thicker in the medial cheek of a female face, whereas the fat distribution is even in a male face [5, 6].

Case Study 6.1

Patient Age: 70
   Sex: Female
   Presenting Concern: Volume loss in cheeks, midcheek groove, palpebromalar groove, tear trough

Grading (before)

- *Midcheek groove*: 4 (severe) (Figure 6.8)
- *Infraorbital hollow*: 4 (very severe) (Figure 6.9)

Treatment Plan

- *Session 1*: Dermal filler using Definisse Restore by Relife to infraorbital region (1.5 ml used in total) and Definisse Core to cheeks and midcheek groove (3 ml used in total) (Figure 6.10)

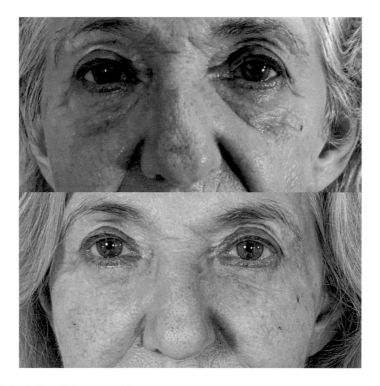

FIGURE 6.8   Patient's frontal view: top and bottom.

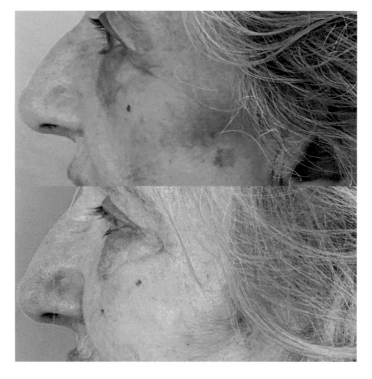

FIGURE 6.9   Patient's frontal view: top and bottom.

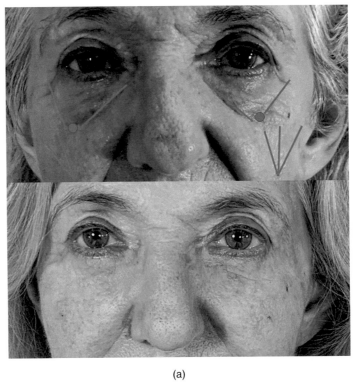

(a)

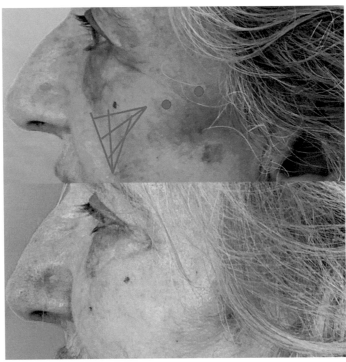

(b)

FIGURE 6.10   (a, b) Straight lines, retrograde linear technique; circle, bolus technique.

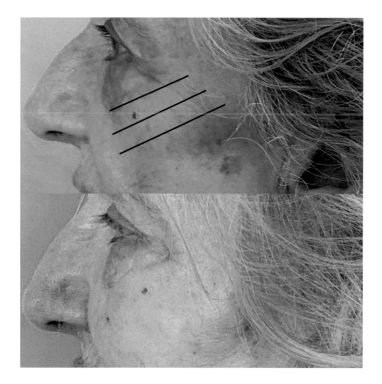

FIGURE 6.11   Straight lines, positioning of threads.

- *Session 2*: Threads using Definisse Free Floating threads by Relife to reposition soft tissue in the cheek area (three threads used per side, six threads in total) (Figure 6.11)
- *Session 3*: Skin peel using Definisse Classic Peel (Figure 6.12)

Grading (after)

- *Midcheek groove*: 0 (none)
- *Infraorbital hollow*: 4 (none)

Case Study 6.2

Patient Age: 40
  Sex: Female
  Presenting Concern: Lack of facial contour and facial asymmetry (Figure 6.13)

Treatment Plan

- *Session 1*: Dermal filler using Definisse Core to cheeks (3 ml used in total) (Figure 6.14)
- *Session 2*: Skin peel using Definisse Classic Peel (Figure 6.15)

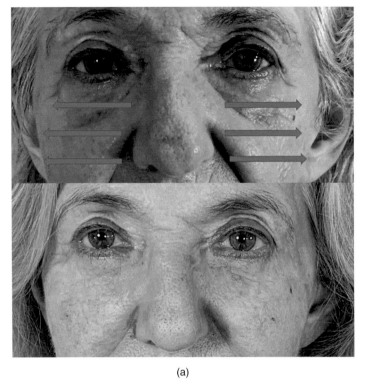

(a)

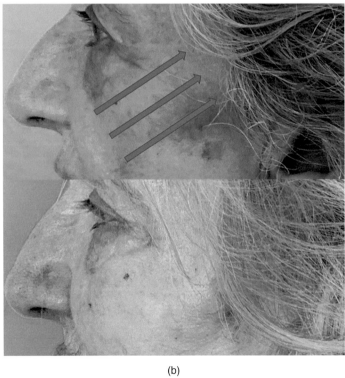

(b)

FIGURE 6.12   (a, b) Arrows, direction of application.

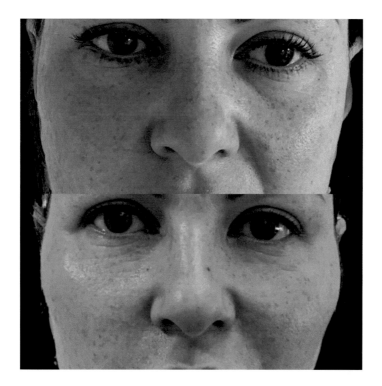

FIGURE 6.13 Patient: top and bottom.

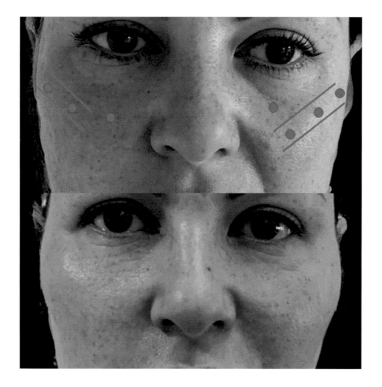

FIGURE 6.14 Straight lines, retrograde linear technique; circle, bolus technique.

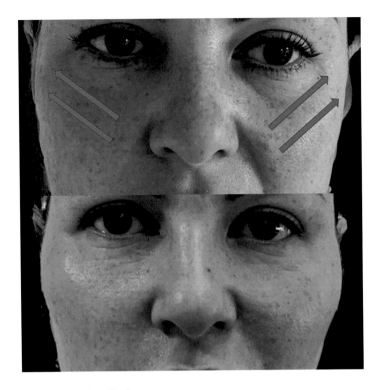

FIGURE 6.15 Arrows, direction of application.

REFERENCES

1. Andre P, Azib N, Berros P, et al. eds. *Anatomy and Volumising Injections.* Paris: E2e Medical Pub.; 2012.
2. Mendelson BC, Jacobson SR, "Surgical anatomy of the midcheek: Facial layers, spaces, and the mid-cheek segments," *Clinics in Plastic Surgery*, vol. 35, no. 3, pp. 395–404, 2008.
3. Salti G, Fundaro SP, "Evaluation of the rheologic and physicochemical properties of a novel hyaluronic acid filler range with eXcellent Three-Dimensional Reticulation (XTR™) technology," *Polymers*, vol. 12, no. 8, p. 1644, 2020.
4. Li Y, Mou S, Xiao P, et al. "Delayed two steps PRP injection strategy for the improvement of fat graft survival with superior angiogenesis," *Scientific Reports*, vol. 10, no. 1, p. 5231, 2020.
5. Wysong A, Kim D, Joseph T, MacFarlane DF, Tang JY, Gladstone HB, "Quantifying soft tissue loss in the aging male face using magnetic resonance imaging," *Dermatologic Surgery*, vol. 40, no. 7, pp. 786–793, 2014.
6. Wysong A, Joseph T, Kim D, Tang JY, Gladstone HB, "Quantifying soft tissue loss in facial aging: A study in women using magnetic resonance imaging," *Dermatologic Surgery*, vol. 39, no. 12, pp. 1895–1902, 2013.

7

The Perioral Region

Vincent Wong

CONTENTS

The perioral region extends from the subnasale to the mentum. The key landmarks for facial aesthetic procedures here are:

- The lips
- Nasolabial folds
- Marionette lines

The perioral region is the most dynamic region of the face and is therefore considered to be one of the most difficult areas to treat. Furthermore, this region also has a complex vasculature – it is essential that the practitioner understands perioral anatomy so that high-risk areas may be identified to prevent serious adverse events from occurring [1]. See Figures 7.1 and 7.2.

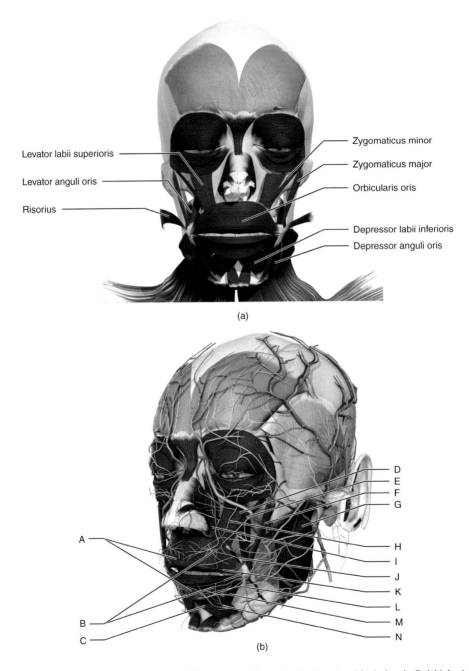

FIGURE 7.1   (a) Muscles of facial expression. (b) Structures of the perioral region: A, orbicularis oris; B, labial vein, superior and inferior branches; C, depressor or labii inferioris; D, levator labii superioris; E, zygomaticus minor; F, zygomaticus major; G, masseter; H, facial nerve, zygomatic branches; I, levator labii superioris alaeque nasi; J, facial nerve, superficial buccal branches; K, labial artery, superior and inferior branches; L, facial nerve, inferior buccal branches; M, facial nerve, inferior mandibular branch; N, inferior alveolar nerve, mental branches. (Adapted from www.anatomy.tv with permission © Informa UK Ltd [trading as Primal Pictures], 2021.)

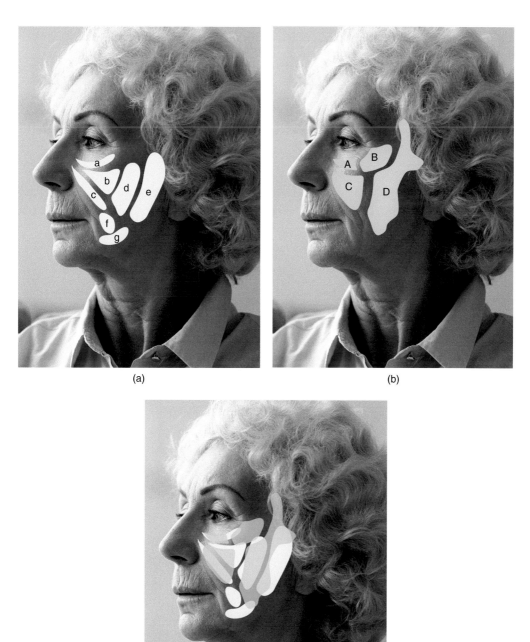

(a)

(b)

(c)

FIGURE 7.2 (a) Superficial cheek fat compartments: a. Infraorbital fat; b, Medial cheek fat; c, Nasolabial fat; d, Middle cheek fat; e, Lateral cheek fat; f, Superior jowl fat; g, Inferior jowl fat. (b) Deep cheek fat compartments: A, Medial sub-orbicularis oculi fat; B, Lateral sub-orbicularis oculi fat; C, Deep medial cheek fat; D, Buccal fat. (c) Superficial and deep cheek fat compartments in relation to each other. (Adapted from Fundarò S, Mauro G, Di Blasio A, et al. [2018] Anatomy and aging of cheek fat compartments, Med Dent Res. 2: DOI: 10.15761/MDR.1000111 under Open Access.)

Lifestyle and external factors also tend to affect this region more, for example, smoking, diet, sun damage, and poor dental health.

Lip Fullness, Perioral Lines, and Gummy Smile

Full and well-defined lips represent attractiveness and beauty, especially on a female face. Changes in lip morphology as a result of ageing include [1, 2]:

- Volume loss and thinning, especially in the upper lip.
- Lipstick bleed line (perioral lines) due to increased muscle tone of orbicularis oris muscle.
- Loss of lip colour resulting in blunt lip margin.
- Lip elongation due to weakening of muscle strength.
- The smile gets narrower vertically and wider transversely showing less maxillary teeth and more mandibular teeth.

Gummy smile is a condition where the patient shows too much gum when smiling. Excessive gingival display occurs when 3 mm or more of gum tissue is exposed when a patient smiles [1, 2]. Some patients are prone to have this kind of smile, such as those with a short distance between the nasal base and Cupid's Bow as well as those with a facial convex profile with a prominent nose and an underdeveloped chin.

Dentistry also plays a significant role in restoring the perioral region, not only in elderly people. Restorative techniques of the perioral soft tissue will further enhance the aesthetic outcome of aesthetic restorative dentistry.

When treating the perioral region, it is important to note that facial characteristics are different in men and women. Men have thinner lips (especially upper lip), larger philtrum widths, and wider mouth width [3].

Rating Scales

- Lip fullness can be assessed using the scale in Figure 7.3.
- The severity of perioral lines can be assessed using the scale in Figure 7.4.

Treatment Options

- Dermal fillers

  Temporary fillers have become the treatment of choice when it comes to lip rejuvenation. Hyaluronic acid (HA) fillers are cross-linked to extend their longevity to 6–12 months.

  Augmenting the perioral region with injectable fillers requires skill and experience to avoid complications and to achieve a natural look. As the lips are very well innervated, topical anaesthesia or nerve block may be used to reduce injection and filling-related pain. Some fillers also contain lidocaine to reduce injection pain. The application of cold compress before and after the procedure can increase patient comfort and help to reduce swelling and tenderness.

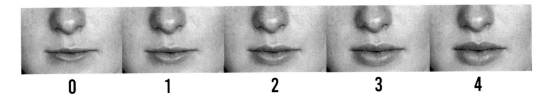

FIGURE 7.3 Lip fullness scale. 0 = very thin, 1 = thin, 2 = moderately thick, 3 = thick, 4 = full (following the scale of Merz Aesthetics).

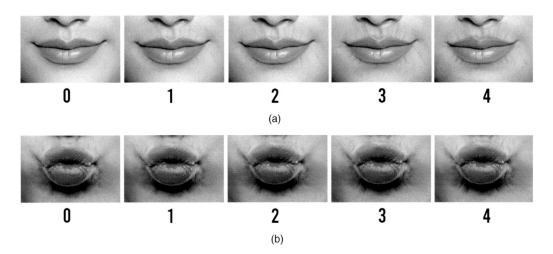

FIGURE 7.4 (a) Perioral wrinkles severity scale (at rest). (b) Perioral wrinkles severity scale (on animation). 0 = no wrinkle, 1 = mild wrinkles, 2 = moderate wrinkles, 3 = severe wrinkles, 4 = very severe wrinkles (following the scales of Merz Aesthetics).

Filling is usually performed in a retrograde manner using linear threading technique; however, bolus and serial puncture techniques are also commonly used depending on the practitioner's preference. Some physicians may prefer cannulas over needles when treating the lips to avoid potential bruising. Regardless of the technique used, injections should always be done slowly to reduce pain and bruising.

Dermal filler injections can be performed in the vermillion border to increase lip definition and to improve the appearance of perioral lines. Injections in the body of the lips can also alter the nasolabial angle by improving the height of lips and lip projection. Strategic placement of fillers can also correct gummy smile as well as enhancing the philtrum and Cupid's bow. In patients with severe perioral lines, dermal fillers may also be injected directly into each line individually using linear threading or serial puncture technique:

- Neurotoxin

As lip lines are caused by increased tone of the orbicularis oris muscle, neurotoxin can help by relaxing the muscle fibres involved. In some patients, the upper lip retracts inwards when smiling despite lip volume – this can also be corrected with neurotoxin by relaxing the relevant muscle fibres (a procedure commonly known as 'lip flip'). Typically, a small amount of neurotoxin is injected in the perioral region (1–2 standardised units per injection, 1–2 injection points per side). If too much neurotoxin is injected, the patient may experience difficulties in speaking and other relevant activities (such as smiling, whistling, and drinking from a straw) due to weakening of muscle fibres.

Within the array of medical aesthetics treatments, neurotoxin is an extremely effective option for correcting gummy smile without altering the volume of the lips [4]. A small dose of neurotoxin (2–4 standardised units) is commonly placed in the Yonsei point, targeting the levator labii superioris, levator labii superioris alaeque nasi, and zygomaticus minor muscles [5]. See Figure 7.5.

- Threads

The use of threads for lip rejuvenation has increased in popularity, especially in Asian countries. Threads are more suited to those wanting subtle to moderate enhancement rather than major revolumisation. The results from thread lift tend to last up to 24 months, which is considerably longer than other available options. Although many types of threads exist, there are barbed threads made of polylactic acid and polycaprolactone that are specially designed for the lips. Apart from repositioning soft tissues (due to the presence of barbs), these threads also have revitalising properties as they stimulate neocollagenesis.

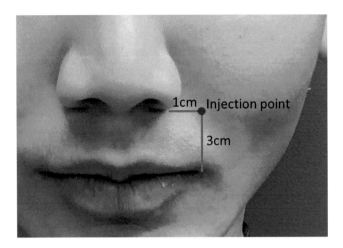

FIGURE 7.5   Yonsei point, measured at 1 cm lateral to ala and 3 cm above the oral commissure.

Combination Treatments

- Combination of neurotoxin and dermal filler
- Combination of neurotoxin and threads
- Combination of neurotoxin, dermal filler, and threads
- Mesotherapy
- Platelet-rich plasma
- Laser resurfacing

Complications

- Bleeding (from needle trauma)
- Nodule formation (over injection of filler)
- Oedema (from needle trauma)
- Bruising (from needle trauma)
- Vascular compromise (from dermal filler injections)
- Necrosis (from dermal filler blocking an artery)
- Infection (from lack of aseptic technique)
- Lip distortion (incorrect placement of neurotoxin)
- Speech impediment (overdose of neurotoxin)
- Granulomas (reactions to dermal filler)
- Skin puckering (from superficial thread placement)

Nasolabial Folds

Nasolabial folds form natural facial contours. However, they can become more prominent with age, projecting a fatigued or drawn appearance. This deepening of the nasolabial folds is due to superficial fat pads undergoing atrophy and redistribution, in addition to bony resorption of the maxilla [6].

A common mistake in correction of the perioral area is usually an error of omission; as nasolabial folds play an important role in ensuring facial balance, leaving this key area out when rejuvenating the perioral region may create an unfinished appearance [3].

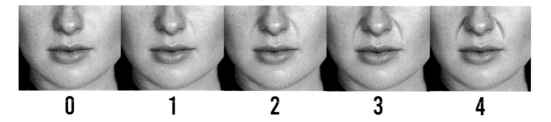

FIGURE 7.6 Nasolabial fold severity scale. 0 = no folds, 1 = mild folds, 2 = moderate folds, 3 = severe folds, 4 = very severe folds (following the scale of Merz Aesthetics).

Rating Scales

The severity of nasolabial fold can be assessed using the scale in Figure 7.6.

Treatment Options

- Dermal fillers

  Understanding the key difference between nasolabial creases and nasolabial folds is important during treatment. Nasolabial creases are skin defects rather than contour deformities, and they appear to be epidermal and dermal (this is more common in younger patients and in patients with thin skin). True nasolabial folds are caused by loss of support and an apparent volume loss.

  When treating nasolabial creases, a filler with mild to moderate viscosity should be injected in the epidermal or dermal layer. For true nasolabial folds, a thicker dermal filler will be necessary (deep dermal or subdermal injections) to restore the facial contour.

  Another method is to augment the cheek itself, which creates a lifting effect and eliminates the nasolabial fold (as discussed in Chapter 6).

- Threads

  Barbed facial threads are highly effective in repositioning soft tissues and superficial fat pads in the cheeks. By elevating the malar fat pad, a softening effect can be seen in the nasolabial folds (as discussed in Chapter 6).

Combination Treatments

- Autologous fat grafting
- Cheek enhancement
- Skin tightening (radiofrequency, ultrasound, fractional laser)

Complications

- Bleeding (from needle trauma)
- Nodule formation (over injection of filler)
- Oedema (from needle trauma)
- Bruising (from needle trauma)
- Vascular compromise (from dermal filler injections)
- Necrosis (from dermal filler blocking an artery)
- Infection (from lack of aseptic technique)
- Granulomas (reactions to dermal filler)
- Skin puckering (from superficial thread placement)

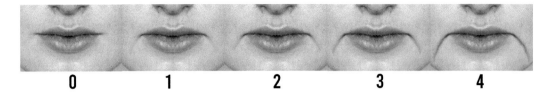

FIGURE 7.7 Marionette fold severity scale. 0 = no folds, 1 = mild folds, 2 = moderate folds, 3 = severe folds, 4 = very severe folds (following the scale of Merz Aesthetics).

Marionette Lines

Commonly known as 'puppet lines', marionette lines (melomental fold) extend from the corners of the mouth to the edge of the mandible. Often, marionette lines are the result of volume loss and contraction of the depressor anguli oris (DAO) muscle. In many cases, marionette lines are paired with a triangular depression below the oral commissure, giving the patient a 'sad look'.

Rating Scale

Marionette lines can be rated according to the scale in Figure 7.7.

Treatment Options

- Dermal filler

  Moderately cross-linked dermal filler can be injected in this region to restore volume. This can be done using a 27G needle or a 25G cannula. Depending on the severity, a mixture of deep (subcutaneous level) and superficial (deep dermis) injections may be required. Dermal filler injections should always be in the middle of the fold and medially to cover the triangular depression below the oral commissure [6].

- Neurotoxin

  In patients with increased DAO tone, the injection of neurotoxin can help correct the downturn of the mouth corners. On average 2–3 units of neurotoxin per side are required. When injecting the DAO, it is important to have the injection site lateral to the marionette line, down at the jaw-line, with the injection being placed deep into the muscle. This will prevent accidental injection into surrounding muscle, especially the depressor anguli inferioris [4].

Combination Treatments

- Neurotoxin and dermal filler
- Lip enhancement
- Midface revolumisation
- Midface tissue repositioning with threads
- Jawline enhancement with dermal filler

Complications

- Oedema (from needle trauma)
- Bruising (from needle trauma)
- Vascular compromise (from dermal filler injections)
- Necrosis (from dermal filler injections blocking an artery)

- Inability to smile/asymmetrical smile (from neurotoxin injection into the wrong muscle)
- Infection (from lack of aseptic technique)

Case Study 7.1

Patient Age: 24
  Sex: Female

Presenting Concern

- Gummy smile and lip volume. The patient does not wish to receive neurotoxin treatment.

Grading (before)

- *Lip fullness*: 1 (thin) (Figure 7.8)

Treatment Plan

- Dermal filler using Definisse Restore by Relife to lips (1 ml used in total) (Figure 7.9)

Grading (after)

- *Lip fullness*: 3 (thick) and elimination of gummy smile

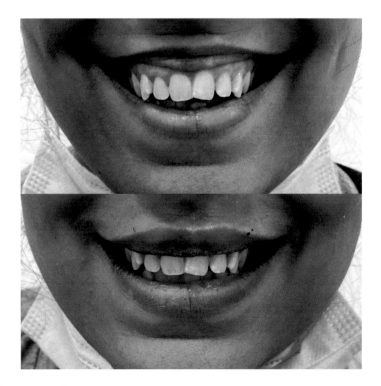

FIGURE 7.8   Patient: top and bottom.

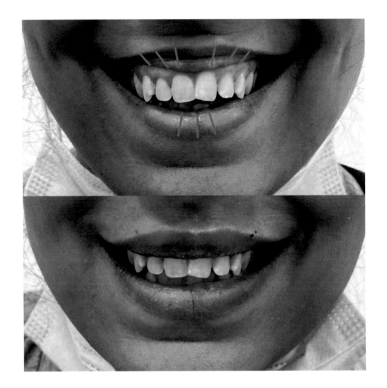

FIGURE 7.9   Straight lines, retrograde linear technique.

Case Study 7.2

Patient Age: 56
  Sex: Female

Presenting Concern

- Lip volume and marionette folds

Grading (before)

- *Lip fullness*: 0 (very thin)
- *Marionette fold:* 3 (severe) (Figure 7.10)

Treatment Plan

- *Session 1*: Dermal filler using Definisse Restore by Relife to lips (1 ml used in total) (Figure 7.11)
- *Session 2*: Dermal filler using Definisse Core by Relife to marionette folds (1 ml used in total) (Figure 7.12)

Grading (after)

- *Lip fullness*: 2 (moderately thick)
- *Marionette fold*: 1 (mild)

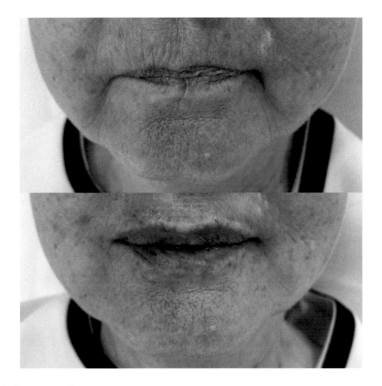

FIGURE 7.10   Patient: top and bottom.

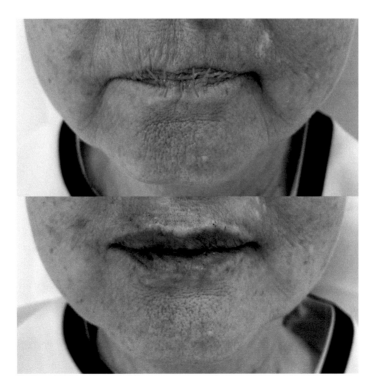

FIGURE 7.11   Straight lines, retrograde linear technique.

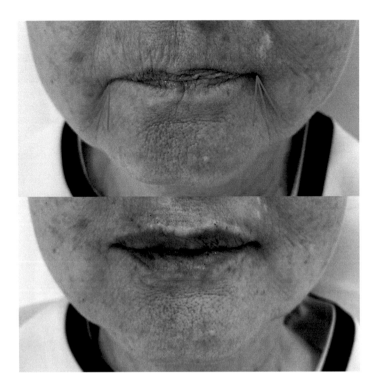

FIGURE 7.12   Straight lines, retrograde linear technique.

Case Study 7.3

Patient Age: 70
  Sex: Female

Presenting Concern

- Nasolabial fold, lip volume, perioral lines, and marionette folds

Grading (before)

- *Lip fullness*: 0 (very thin)
- *Marionette fold*: 4 (very severe)
- *Nasolabial fold*: 4 (very severe)
- *Perioral lines*: 4 (very severe) (Figure 7.13)

Treatment Plan

- *Session 1*: Dermal filler using Definisse Restore by Relife to lips and philtrum (1 ml used in total), and Definisse Core to cheeks, nasolabial folds, and marionette folds (6 ml used in total) (Figure 7.14)
- *Session 2*: Botulinum toxin using Botox by Allergan to perioral lines (8 units used in total) (Figure 7.15)
- *Session 3*: Threads using Definisse Free Floating threads by Relife to reposition soft tissue in the cheek area (three threads used per side, six threads in total) (Figure 7.16)
- *Session 4*: Skin peel using Definisse Classic Peel (Figure 7.17)

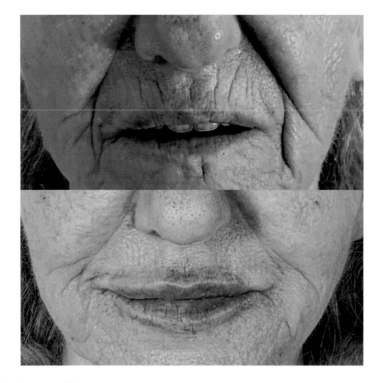

FIGURE 7.13 Patient: top and bottom.

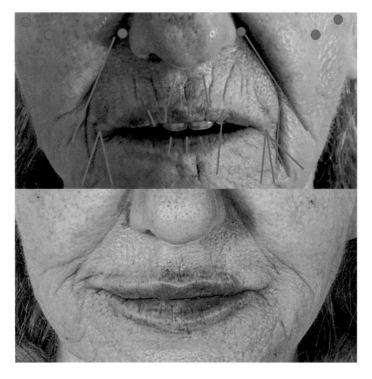

FIGURE 7.14 Straight lines, retrograde linear technique; circles, bolus technique.

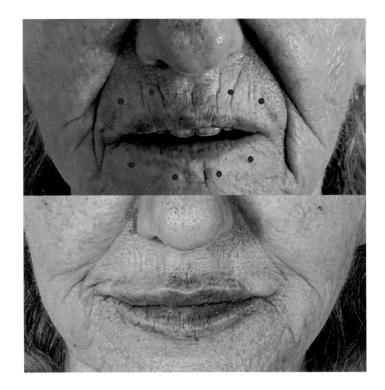

FIGURE 7.15   Red dots, 1 u of botulinum toxin.

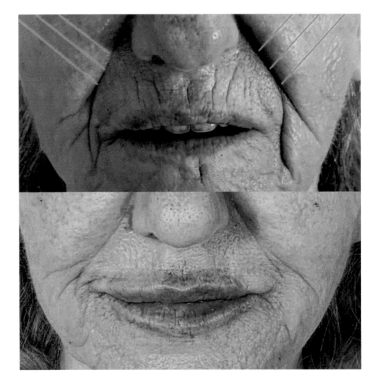

FIGURE 7.16   Straight lines, positioning of threads.

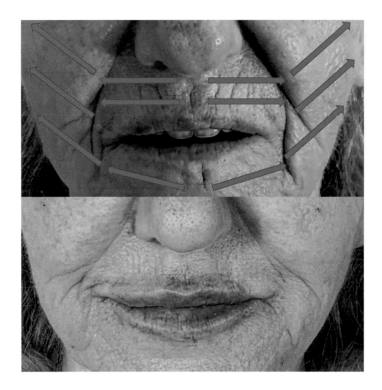

FIGURE 7.17 Arrows, direction of peel application.

Grading (after)

- *Lip fullness*: 2 (moderately thick)
- *Marionette fold*: 1 (mild)
- *Nasolabial fold*: 2 (moderate)
- *Perioral lines*: 2 (moderate)

REFERENCES

1. Hotta TA, "Understanding the perioral anatomy," *Plastic Surgical Nursing*, vol. 36, no. 1, pp. 12–18, 2016.
2. Wollina U, "Perioral rejuvenation: Restoration of attractiveness in aging females by minimally invasive procedures," *Clinical Interventions in Aging*, vol. 8, no. 1, pp. 1149–1155, 2018.
3. Farhadian JA, Bloom BS, Brauer JA, "Male aesthetics: A review of facial anatomy and pertinent clinical implications," *Journal of Drugs in Dermatology*, vol. 14, no. 9, pp. 1029–34, 2015.
4. Cohen JL, Ozog DM, eds. *Botulinum Toxins: Cosmetic and Clinical Applications. Treatment of the Perioral Area*. Hoboken, NJ: John Wiley & Sons Ltd; 2017.
5. Lova F, Ahsan A, "Botox – the magical spell of dentistry: A literature review," *Manipal Journal of Dental Sciences*, vol. 3, no. 1, pp. 31–36, 2018.
6. Andre P, Azib N, Berros P, et al. eds. *Anatomy and Volumising Injections*. Paris: E2e Medical Pub.; 2012.

8

The Chin

Vincent Wong

CONTENTS

The chin forms the lower topographic limit of the face and plays a crucial role in the perception of attractiveness. When it comes to facial balance and harmony, the chin must be assessed in both frontal and profile views.

Facial attractiveness is characterised by a combination of factors that involve symmetry and proportions that are deemed aesthetically pleasing. From the front, the face can be divided into horizontal thirds that are equal in height. Hence, a vertically deficient (microgenia) or excessive chin (macrogenia) places the lower third of the face out of balance when compared to the middle and upper thirds of the face [1]. Similarly, in profile view, horizontal deficiency (retrogenia or retrognathia) or excess (mandibular prognathism) diminishes facial harmony [1].

Apart from the aforementioned proportions, the chin also has an important role in the appreciation of other facial features [1]. For example, a large nose is often paired with a deficient chin. As they have a reciprocally negative effect on the appearance of each other as well as the overall facial attractiveness, chin enhancement usually takes the focus away from the otherwise prominent nose [1, 2].

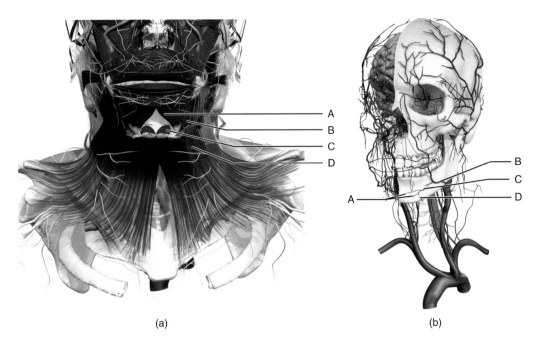

(a)   (b)

FIGURE 8.1 (a) Muscles affecting the chin: A, depressor labii inferioris; B, depressor anguli oris; C, mentalis; D, platysma. (b) Vasculature of the chin: A, mental artery (terminal branches of inferior alveolar artery arising from external maxillary artery); B, external maxillary artery; C, inferior alveolar artery; D, submental artery. (Adapted from www.anatomy.tv with permission © Informa UK Ltd [trading as Primal Pictures], 2021.)

Sexual dimorphism (the phenotypic differences between the sexes) is often more obvious in the lower face. Hence it is of utmost importance that we have a profound appreciation of male and female beauty. The chin is usually larger and more protruding in men, with well-developed lateral tubercle – whereas a female chin is smaller, narrower and more pointed [3]. See Figure 8.1.

Chin Deficiency and Reshaping

Chin deficiency can be further divided into vertical and horizontal dimensions.

Assessment of Vertical Dimension

The lower third of the face (subnasale to menton) can be further divided using a horizontal line passing through the stomion. The distance between stomion to menton should be twice the distance between subnasale to stomion in a harmonious face [1, 2, 4]. See Figure 8.2.

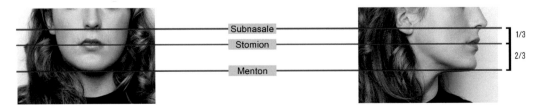

FIGURE 8.2 Assessment and proportions of the lower third of the face.

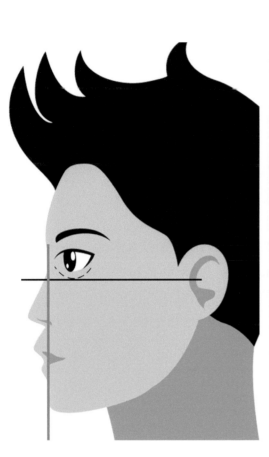

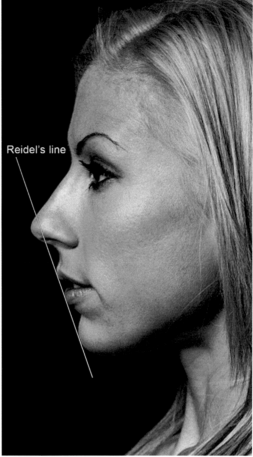

FIGURE 8.3 Assessment of chin projection using Frankfort horizontal.

FIGURE 8.4 Reidel's plane.

Assessment of Horizontal Dimension

Horizontal assessment of the chin is best done in profile. This can be done with the patient's head positioned in such a way that a line connecting the superior aspect of the auditory canal to the orbital margin lies parallel to the floor (Frankfort horizontal) [1]. In this position, a vertical line from the nasion should cross the horizontal plane at 90 degrees (right angle), and the pogonion should touch this line [1]. In patients with retrogenia or retrognathia, the chin lies behind this line; the chin will cross this line in those with mandibular prognathism. See Figure 8.3.

Another way to assess the horizontal projection of the chin is by using Reidel's plane – if the ideal chin projection is present, the most projecting portion of the upper lip, lower lip and chin (pogonion) would all be tangent to the same line [1]. Retrogenia or retrognathia is present when the pogonion lies posterior to the Riedel's plane (Figure 8.4).

Rating Scale

The rating scales in Figure 8.5 can be used in clinical assessment to determine the extent of chin deficiency.

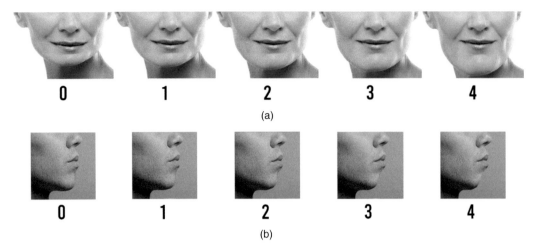

FIGURE 8.5 (a) Vertical chin height assessment scale. 0 = severely deficient, 1 = mildly deficient, 2 = ideal chin height, 3 = mildly excessive, 4 = severely excessive. (b) Horizontal chin projection scale. 0 = ideal projection, 1 = mild deficient, 2 = moderate deficient, 3 = severe deficient, 4 = very severe deficient.

Treatment Option

- Dermal filler

  Strategic placement of dermal fillers can help patients with chin deficiency to achieve facial balance and harmony. Furthermore, those with asymmetry and those who would like to change the shape of their chin could also benefit from this treatment. An ideal dermal filler for this region would be cross-linked with a high G′ (lifting capacity) so that projection or elongation can be achieved with minimal amount of product [4]. Apart from injections in the mental crease (subcutaneous layer), injections in the chin should be performed deep, right on the periosteum level. When injecting the anterior chin, it is important to keep injection points in the medial aspect to avoid the mental artery [5].

Combination Treatments

- Neurotoxin (see below)
- Dermal fillers in the jawline and marionette lines

Complications

- Oedema (from needle trauma)
- Bruising (from needle trauma)
- Vascular compromise
- Necrosis
- Infection (from lack of aseptic technique)

Chin Dimpling

A dimpled chin (sometimes referred to as 'golf ball chin' or 'peau d'orange') is a result of an overactive mentalis. This is often exacerbated by chin movements. Although chin dimpling can be caused by volume loss and chronological ageing, the most common cause is genetic inheritance.

Treatment Option

- Neurotoxin

  Dimpling of the chin can be improved greatly with neurotoxin injection into the mentalis [6]. Usually, 2–5 standardised units are required depending of the extent of dimpling. With careful placement in the midline, the mentalis muscle can be sufficiently relaxed so that the surface area becomes smooth while maintaining natural movements [6].

Combination Treatment

- Dermal filler for deeper dimpling

Complications

- Oedema (from needle trauma)
- Bruising (from needle trauma)
- Paralysis of the chin (from high dosage of neurotoxin)
- Infection (from lack of aseptic technique)

Case Study 8.1

Patient Age: 40
  Sex: Female

Presenting Concern

- *Asymmetrical lips*: The patient would like fuller lips, too.
- Deficiency in chin height and the patient would like to change her chin shape to become pointier.

Grading (before)

- *Vertical chin height*: 1 (mildly deficient)
- *Lip fullness scale*: 2 (moderately thick) (Figure 8.6)

Treatment Plan

- Dermal filler to lips using Definisse Touch by Relife (1 ml used), followed by dermal filler to chin using Definisse Core by Relife (2 ml used) (Figure 8.7)

Grading (after)

- Vertical chin height: 2 (ideal chin height)
- Lip fullness scale: 4 (full)
- Lip symmetry and a pointy chin were also achieved

Case Study 8.2

Patient Age: 35
  Sex: Male

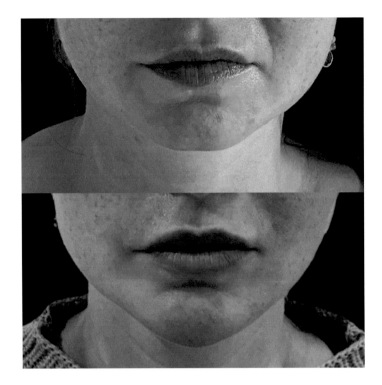

FIGURE 8.6   Patient: top and bottom.

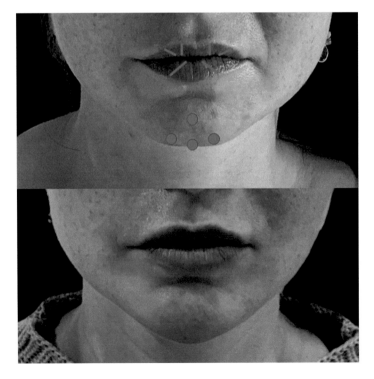

FIGURE 8.7   Straight line, retrograde linear technique; circle, bolus technique.

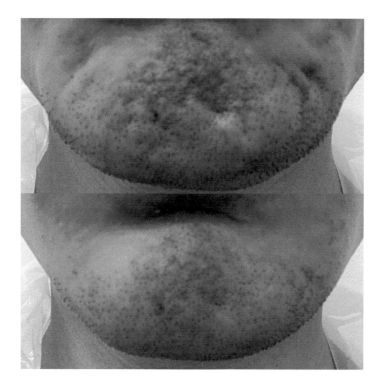

FIGURE 8.8   Patient: top and bottom.

Presenting Concern

- Chin dimpling (Figure 8.8)

Treatment Plan

- Neurotoxin to mentalis muscle using Botox by Allergan (four units used) (Figure 8.9)

Result

- Reduction in chin dimpling

Case Study 8.3

Patient Age: 20
  Sex: Transgender male

Presenting Concern

- Rounded and feminine-looking chin. The patient started hormone therapy (testosterone) 6 months prior to appointment and would like to achieve a squarer and more masculine-looking chin (Figure 8.10).

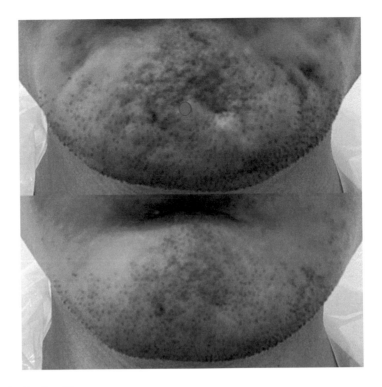

FIGURE 8.9   Blue dot, 4 u of Botox.

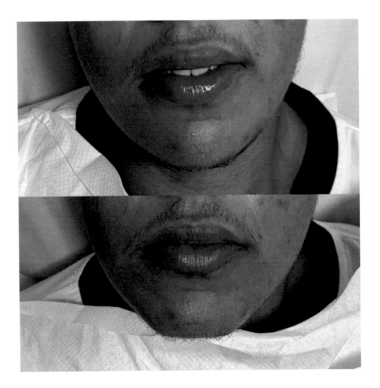

FIGURE 8.10   Patient: top and bottom.

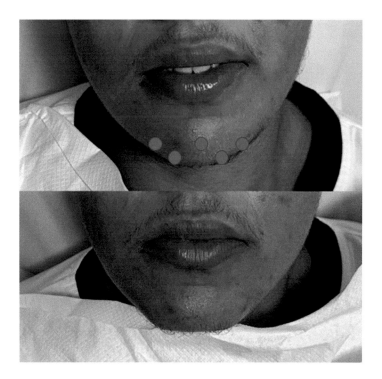

FIGURE 8.11 Circle, bolus technique.

Treatment Plan

- Dermal filler to chin using Juvederm Volux by Allergan (3 ml used) (Figure 8.11)

Result

- Masculine chin with well-defined lateral tubercles

REFERENCES

1. Guyuron B, Weinfeld AB, "Genioplasty," *Plastic Reconstructive Surgery*, Clinicalgate.com, 2015.
2. Ahmed J, Patil S, Jayaraj S, "Assessment of the chin in patients undergoing rhinoplasty: What proportion may benefit from chin augmentation?," *Otolaryngology – Head and Neck Surgery*, vol. 142, no. 2, pp. 164–168, 2010.
3. Ravichandran E, Ravichandran S, "Male vs. female facial rejuvenation," *Aesthetics Journal*, vol. 2, no. 11, 2015.
4. Sykes JM, Fitzgerald R, "Choosing the best procedure to augment the chin: Is anything better than an implant?," *Facial Plastic Surgery*, vol. 35, no. 2, pp. 507–512, 2016.
5. Fang M, Rahman E, Kapoor KM, "Managing complications of submental artery involvement after hyaluronic acid filler injection in chin region," *Plastic and Reconstructive Surgery Global Open*, vol. 6, no. 5, 2018.
6. Beer K, Yohn M, Closter J, "A double-blinded, placebo-controlled study of Botox for the treatment of subjects with chin rhytids," *Journal of Drugs in Dermatology*, vol. 4, no. 4, pp. 417–422, 2005.

9

The Jawline and Neck

Vincent Wong

CONTENTS

The structure of the lower third of the face contributes significantly to a youthful and harmonious appearance. The ageing process of the lower jawline and neck comprises [1]:

- Atrophy of deep and superficial fat
- Dehiscence of the mandibular septum
- Increased muscle tone, especially the platysma muscle
- Increase in skin laxity

This combination leads to downward migration of both fat compartments towards the neck. Combined with age-related bone resorption and remodelling (starting from age 35), this results in a loss of mandibular height and length, a more obtuse mandibular angle, chin retrusion, and an accentuated pre-jowl sulcus [2]. On the surface, this presents as melomental folds, deep mental crease, double chin, jowls, and poorly defined jawline [2]. See Figure 9.1.

Jowl and Jawline Remodelling

Jowls are a common sign of ageing and are characterised by sagging soft tissue just under the jawline. The appearance of jowls is often paired with loss of jawline definition and chin deficiency [1, 2]. Therefore, anterior, lateral, and dynamic assessment of the lower face should be performed before treatment.

The severity of jowls can be categorised using the scale in Figure 9.2.

Treatment Options

- Dermal filler

   The aim of dermal filler treatment in the jawline would be to help restore lost volume and recreate jawline definition, including enhancing the angle of the mandible. By adding volume to the jawline, it will help reduce the appearance of sagginess by holding the soft tissue better [3]. In order to achieve this, a highly cross-linked hyaluronic acid filler is preferred, although dermal fillers of other origins (calcium hydroxyapetite and polycaprolactone) are also suitable [3]. Usually 3–4 ml of dermal fillers would be required to achieve satisfactory results. Injections can be performed using 25G cannula or 27G needle. The areas that need to be addressed include [4]:

   a. *Pre-auricular area:* Injections here should be in the lateral temporal fat compartment (subcutaneous layer).

   b. *Mandible angle:* For a male patient, injection should be at the supraperiosteal level to widen the face. For a female patient, injections should be more superficial in the subcutaneous layer in order to define the mandible angle.

   c. *Mandible body:* Injections along the mandible body should be in the subcutaneous layer in order to create a defined jawline in young patients (supraperiosteal injections if restoring jawline definition in older patients). Care must be taken to avoid the facial artery, which is located immediately adjacent to the anterior border of the masseter muscle. In some occasions, a mixture of superficial and deep injections is required to achieve the best aesthetic outcome.

   d. *Pre-jowl sulcus:* This is the area immediately anterior to the jowl. Injections here should be deep in the supraperiosteal level.

- Threads

   Ptotic soft tissue can be repositioned with the help of facial threads, which can be made of different materials with varying longevity. For the jawline area, convergent bidirectional threads have proven to be effective [5]. These threads are usually between 16 and 23 cm in

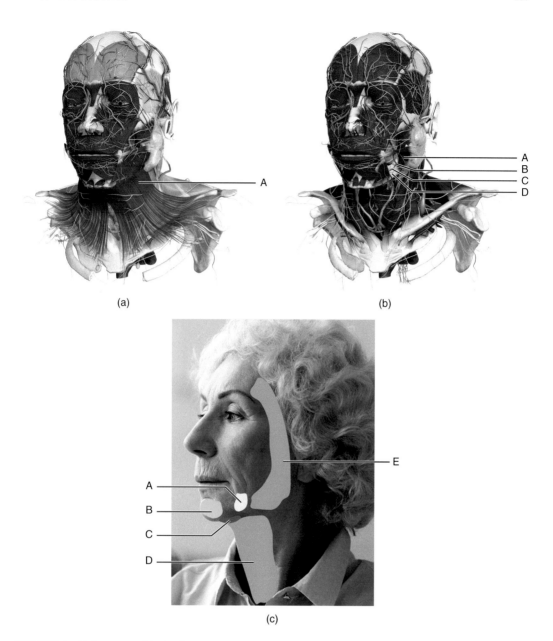

(a)

(b)

(c)

FIGURE 9.1 (a) Structures of the jawline: A, platysma. (b) Structures of the jawline: A, masseter; B, facial vein; C, facial artery; D, mandible. (a,b: Adapted from www.anatomy.tv with permission © Informa UK Ltd [trading as Primal Pictures], 2021.) (c) Fat pads affecting the jawline and neck: A, inferior jowl; B, premental; C, submental; D, pre-platysmal; E, lateral temporal cheek.

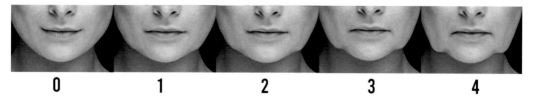

FIGURE 9.2 Jowl severity scale. 0 = no jowls, 1 = mild jowls, 2 = moderate jowls, 3 = severe jowls, 4 = very severe jowls (following the scale of Merz Aesthetics).

length and generally consist of two needles (one at either end of the thread). The barbs (or cones in some cases) work to secure soft tissue in the subcutaneous layer so that they can be repositioned when the thread is lifted and pulled. The most widely used technique is an L-shaped placement of the thread; one end of the thread will be anchored to the pre-auricular/temporal region where the subcutaneous tissue is more fixated and tethered to deeper layers, while the other end of the thread works to hold the more mobile subcutaneous tissue along the jawline. Using a similar concept, V-shaped thread placement can also be used. See Figure 9.3.

Combination of Treatments

- Combination of neuromodulator, threads, and filler
- Chin treatment
- Midface enhancement

Complications

- Venous compression and/or necrosis (from vascular occlusion from dermal fillers)
- Extensive swelling (from needle trauma)
- Extensive bruising (from needle trauma)
- Skin puckering (from thread treatments, some cases may require mechanical release and/or thread removal)
- Fibrosis (scar tissue formation as a reaction to thread as a foreign body)
- Infection (from lack of aseptic technique)

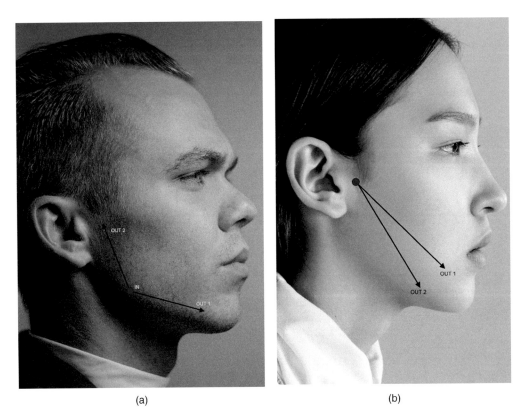

(a)   (b)

FIGURE 9.3   L- and V-shaped thread placement in the lower face.

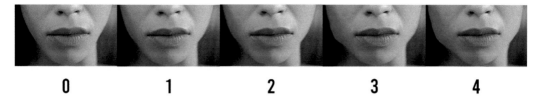

FIGURE 9.4 Masseter thickness assessment scale. 0 = no masseter thickness, 1 = mild masseter thickness, 2 = moderate masseter thickness, 3 = severe masseter thickness, 4 = very severe masseter thickness.

Overactive Masseter and 'Jawline Slimming'

The masseter muscle is a powerful superficial quadrangular muscle originating from the zygomatic arch and inserts along the angle and lateral surface of the mandibular ramus [2]. It is one of the muscles of mastication, and its main function is to elevate the mandible (during the closing of the mouth/jaw and clenching). In some patients, especially those who grind their teeth during sleep, this muscle can be overactive. Asian patients are also more prone to having overactive masseter muscles. The superficial fibres of masseter can cause protrusion, resulting in a square jaw and wider face.

The severity of overactive masseter can be assessed using the rating scale in Figure 9.4.

Treatment Options

- Neurotoxin

    The bulk of masseter can be reduced using neurotoxin. By relaxing the muscle, we can effectively reduce the thickness of it, resulting in a slimmer looking face (more V-shaped) and some relief from the symptoms of teeth grinding. Usually at least 10–25 units of neurotoxin are required per side.

Combination of Treatments

- Neuromodulator treatment for the neck
- Jawline enhancement with dermal filler

Complications

- Swelling (from needle trauma)
- Bruising (from needle trauma)
- Weak bite (from overdose of neurotoxin)
- Infection (from lack of aseptic technique)

Neck Bands

Neck bands can be divided into horizontal and vertical bands. They are caused by the combination of [2]:

a. Increase in skin laxity (and lack of skin structure)
b. Increase in muscle tone
c. Muscle atrophy and soft tissue volume lost

Treatment Options

- Neurotoxin

    Neurotoxins are particularly useful in vertical neck bands, as they are mainly caused by increased platysmal tone. Injections of two standardised units of neurotoxin, directly into the band itself, should be repeated along the band at a distance of 1–1.5 cm between the injection points. In some cases, injections may have to be extended along the inferior border of the mandible, to target platysma fibres that insert into the skin and subcutaneous tissue of the lower face.

- Dermal filler

    Uncrosslinked and lightly cross-linked hyaluronic acid dermal fillers can help soften the appearance of horizontal neck bands. Injections should be placed superficially in the dermis, using retrograde or serial puncture technique. Such injections will also increase hydration of the treatment area.

- Threads

    Threads (as discussed above) may also be used effectively in the neck region in selected patients where tissue repositioning is required [6]. Depending on the presentation, threads are usually inserted under the mandible and anchored behind the ears, or in a 'zigzag' pattern with anchor points along the mandible. The treatment works better after neurotoxin treatment to the neck.

Combination of Treatments

- Combination of neurotoxin, dermal fillers, and threads
- Jawline enhancement with dermal filler
- Masseter reduction with neurotoxin
- Chin enhancement
- Fat dissolving injections for submental fat

Complications

- Difficulty swallowing (from overdosing of neurotoxin)
- Neck weakness when animated (from overdosing of neurotoxin)
- Extensive swelling (from needle trauma)
- Extensive bruising (from needle trauma)
- Skin puckering (from thread treatments, some cases may require mechanical release and/or thread removal)
- Fibrosis (scar tissue formation as a reaction to thread as a foreign body)
- Infection (from lack of aseptic technique)

Submental Fat

Often referred to as a 'double chin', submental fat is often associated with weight gain but can also be inherited [7]. In some patients, skin laxity in the jawline and chin area can also exacerbate the appearance of submental fat.

The severity of submental fat is best assessed in profile, and the rating scale in Figure 9.5 can be used in clinical assessment.

Treatment Options

- Fat dissolving injection

    The active ingredient in fat dissolving injections is deoxycholic acid, a secondary bile acid that helps with emulsification of fat [7]. When injected in small volumes directly into the fat tissue,

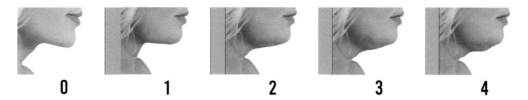

FIGURE 9.5 Submental fat assessment scale. 0 = no submental fat, 1 = mild submental fat, 2 = moderate submental fat, 3 = severe submental fat, 4 = very severe submental fat.

deoxycholic acid disrupts the fat tissue by dissolving the membranes of adipocytes. The resulting glycerol and fatty acids are excreted through the lymphatic system. Whilst the body can regenerate fat cells, the process is very slow. Hence, the results from deoxycholic acid injections can last for an extended period of time, as long as the patient continues to maintain a healthy lifestyle.

Combination of Treatments

- Threads in the neck area
- Jawline enhancement with dermal filler
- Chin enhancement
- HIFU

Complications

- Extensive swelling (from needle trauma and reaction to deoxycholic acid)
- Extensive bruising (from needle trauma)
- Itchiness in the treated area (from reaction to deoxycholic acid)
- Infection (from lack of aseptic technique)
- Nerve injury (from needle trauma and reaction to deoxycholic acid)
- Alopecia at injection site (from reaction to deoxycholic acid)

Case Study 9.1

Patient Age: 35
  Sex: Male

Presenting Concern

- Overactive masseter with teeth grinding

Grading (before)

- *Masseter thickness:* 4 (very severe) (Figure 9.6)

Treatment Plan

- Botulinum toxin using Botox by Allergan (25 units to masseter on each side, 50 units in total) (Figure 9.7)

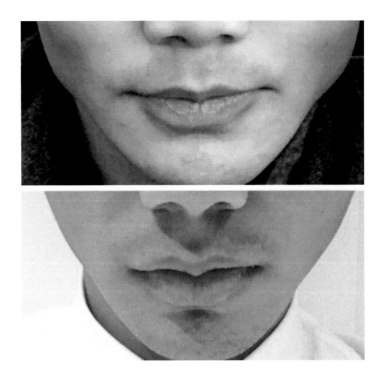

FIGURE 9.6   Patient: top and bottom.

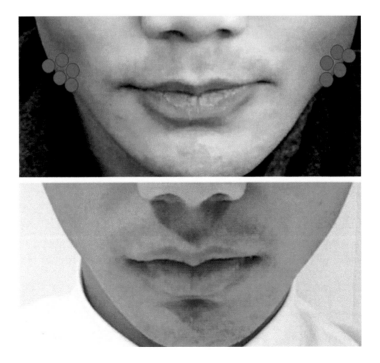

FIGURE 9.7   Blue dot, 5 u.

Grading (after)

- *Masseter thickness:* Grade 0 (none)

Case Study 9.2

Patient Age: 48
  Sex: Female

Presenting Concern

- Vertical neck bands
- Loss of jawline definition (Figure 9.8)

Treatment Plan

- *Session 1:* Botulinum toxin using Botox by Allergan to the neck (30 units in total) (Figure 9.9)
- *Session 2:* Thread lift using Definisse Double Needle thread by Relife (Figure 9.10)

Result

- Smoother appearance of neck and well-defined jawline

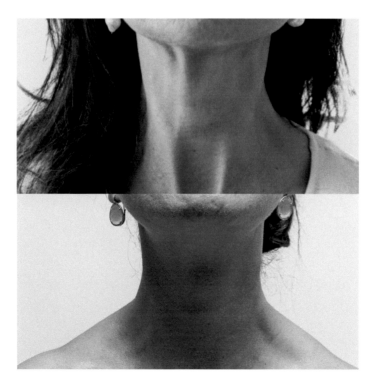

FIGURE 9.8   Patient: top and bottom.

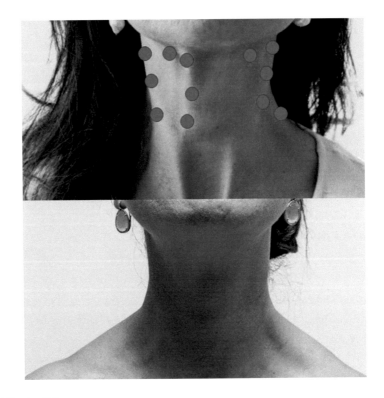

FIGURE 9.9   Blue dot, 2.5 u.

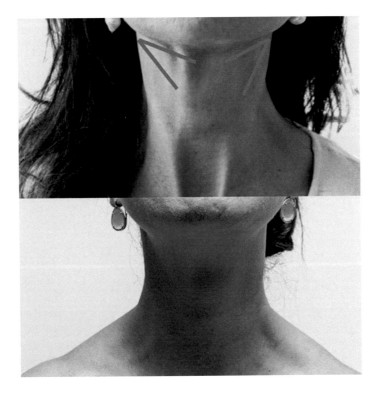

FIGURE 9.10   Straight line, thread placement.

Case Study 9.3

Patient Age: 40
  Sex: Female

Presenting Concern

- Appearance of jowls and lack of jawline definition
- Appearance of double chin
- Retrogenia

Grading (before)

- *Jowl severity:* 1 (mild)
- *Horizontal chin projection:* 2 (moderate deficiency)
- *Submental fat:* 3 (severe) (Figure 9.11)

Treatment Plan

- Dermal fillers using Definisse Core by Relife to mandible, chin, pre-jowl sulcus and cheeks (7 ml used in total) (Figure 9.12)

Grading (after)

- *Jowl severity:* 0 (none)
- *Horizontal chin projection:* 0 (ideal)
- *Submental fat:* 0 (none – corrected by restructuring chin and jawline with dermal fillers)

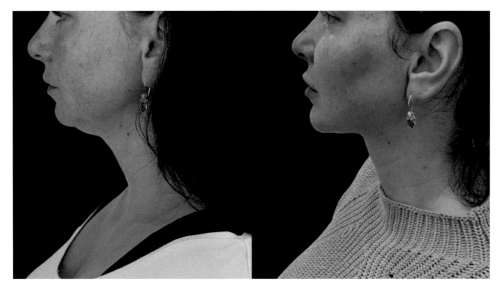

FIGURE 9.11   Patient: top and bottom.

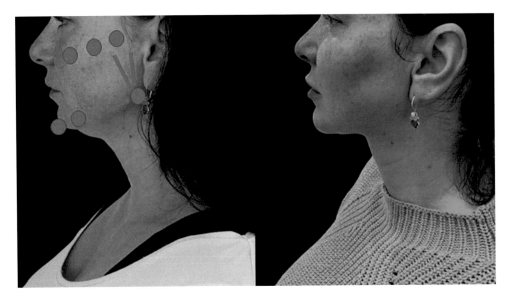

FIGURE 9.12   Straight line, retrograde linear technique; circle, bolus technique.

Case Study 9.4

Patient Age: 51
   Sex: Female

Presenting Concern

- Ptosis of soft tissue in the neck and submental area (Figure 9.13)

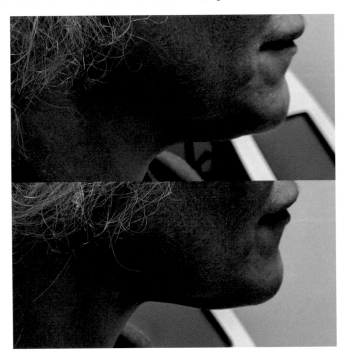

FIGURE 9.13   Patient: top and bottom.

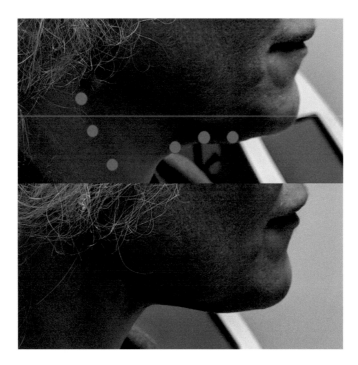

FIGURE 9.14 Blue dot, 2.5 u.

Treatment Plan

- *Session 1:* Botulinum toxin using Botox by Allergan to the neck (30 units in total) (Figure 9.14)
- *Session 2:* Thread lift using Definisse Double Needle thread by Relife (Figure 9.15)

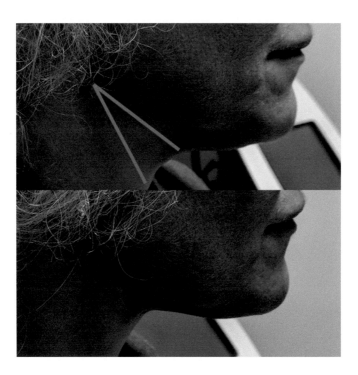

FIGURE 9.15 Straight line, thread placement.

Result

- Improvement of cervicomental angle

Case Study 9.5

Patient Age: 31
  Sex: Female

Presenting Concern

- Presence of submental fat

Grading (before)

- *Submental fat:* 4 (very severe) (Figure 9.16)

Treatment Plan

- Fat dissolving injections with Celluform Plus by Promoitalia (two sessions, one month apart) (Figure 9.17)

Grading (after)

- *Submental fat:* 2 (moderate)

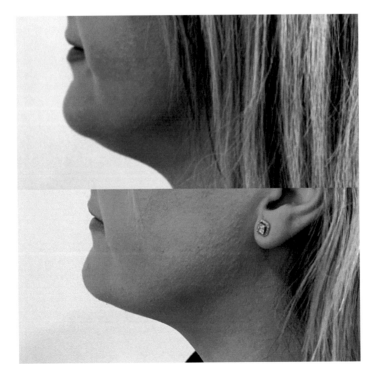

FIGURE 9.16   Patient: top and bottom.

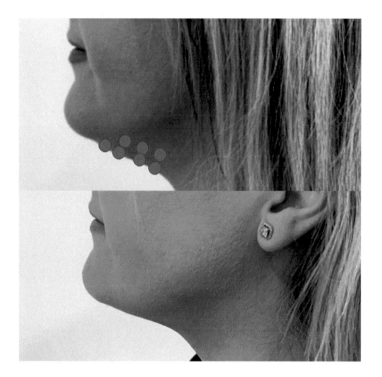

FIGURE 9.17 Blue dot, injection sites.

REFERENCES

1. Coleman S, Grover R, "The anatomy of the aging face: Volume loss and changes in 3-dimensional topography," *Aesthetic Surgery Journal*, vol. 26, no. 1, pp. 4–9, 2006.
2. Agarwal A, DeJoseph L, Silver W, "Anatomy of the jawline, neck, and perioral area with clinical correlations," *Facial Plastic Surgery*, vol. 21, no. 1, pp. 3–10, 2005.
3. Moradi A, Shirazi A, David R, "Nonsurgical chin and jawline augmentation using calcium hydroxylapatite and hyaluronic acid fillers," *Facial Plastic Surgery*, vol. 35, no. 2, pp. 140–148, 2019.
4. Vazirnia A, Braz A, Fabi SG, "Nonsurgical jawline rejuvenation using injectable fillers," *Journal of Cosmetic Dermatology*, vol. 19, no. 8, pp. 1940–1947, 2020.
5. Khiabanloo SR, Jebreili R, Aalipour E, Saljoughi N, Shahidi A, "Outcomes in thread lift for face and neck: A study performed with Silhouette Soft and Promo Happy Lift double needle, innovative and classic techniques," *Journal of Cosmetic Dermatology*, vol. 18, no. 1, pp. 84–93, 2018.
6. Kaminer MS, Bogart M, Choi C, Wee SA, "Long-term efficacy of anchored barbed sutures in the face and neck," *Dermatologic Surgery*, vol. 34, no. 8, pp. 1041–1047, 2008.
7. Shridharani S, Behr K, "ATX-101 (deoxycholic acid injection) treatment in men: Insights from our clinical experience," *Dermatologic Surgery*, vol. 43, no. 1, pp. 225–230, 2017.

10

The Scalp

Kelly Morrell, Naomi O'Hara Collins, and Vincent Wong

CONTENTS

Hair is made up of a protein called keratin and is produced by keratinocytes in hair follicles found in the dermis. As follicles produce new hair cells, older cells are pushed through the surface of the scalp at a rate of approximately six inches per year. The hair visible to the eye is actually a string of dead keratin cells. The average number of hair on an adult head ranges between 100,000 and 150,000 with an average loss of 100 per day.

At any one time, approximately 90% of hair is growing as the hair follicles would be at different stages of the hair cycle. The hair cycle consists of three main phases (Figure 10.1) [1]:

1. *Anagen*: Active hair growth that lasts between 2 and 6 years.
2. *Catagen*: Transitional hair growth that lasts 2–3 weeks.
3. *Telogen*: Resting phase that lasts between 2 and 3 months; at the end of telogen, the hair is shed, and a new hair replaces it – and the growing cycle starts again.

Hair Loss and Hair Thinning

Hair growth and quality of hair can be greatly affected by scalp health – damaged or miniaturised hair follicles cannot efficiently produce hair and will eventually die. Careful consideration to the selection of cleansing and styling products is important to the health of the scalp as certain ingredients can be toxic [1]. Hair follicles can also be damaged by chemical processing, poor nutrition, stress, environmental hazards, chlorine, and certain medications [1, 2].

The main types of alopecia include [1, 2]:

1. *Involutional alopecia* (shortened growth phase, thinning hair follicles, capillary collapse resulting in insufficient nutrients)
2. *Androgenic alopecia* (miniaturisation of hair follicles induced by androgens, defect in conversion of hair follicle stem cells to progenitor cells)
3. *Alopecia areata* (autoimmune disorder, with the presence of cytokines that inhibit hair growth)
4. *Telogen effluvium* (premature termination of anagen phase)
5. *Scarring alopecia* (scar tissue destroys hair follicles and the ability to regenerate)

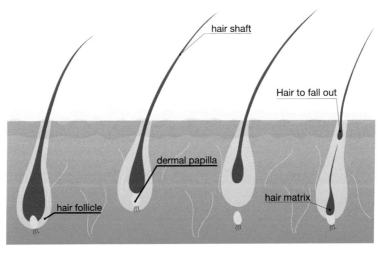

FIGURE 10.1 The hair cycle.

Techniques used for hair and scalp examination can be divided into three categories [2]:

a. Non-invasive methods
  - For example, clinical history, general examination, hair count, weighing shed hair, pull test, trichoscopy, and laser scanning microscopy
b. Semi-invasive methods
  - For example, trichogram, where 60–80 hairs are plucked from a 5-day unwashed hair and immediately placed on a glass slide in an embedding medium to analyse for information on the state of the root (proximal end of hair shaft), the tip, and hair root
c. Invasive methods
  - For example, biopsies for scarring alopecia

The course of treatment for hair loss and hair thinning is heavily dependent on the availability of viable hair follicles. If hair follicles are present, treatments tend to be geared towards follicle stimulation, nourishment, and progression. In cases where hair follicles are not present or have been destroyed (e.g. scarring alopecia), the aims of treatments would be to replace hair follicles (e.g. hair transplant), camouflage the area, or a mixture of both.

Non-surgical interventions have been shown to be successful in involutional alopecia, androgenic alopecia, and telogen effluvium due to availability of active hair follicles. Prior to treatment, an assessment with a handheld trichoscope should be used to confirm the presence of active hair follicles in the treatment area.

Severity Assessment

For men, the Norwood scale is most often used (Figure 10.2).

Stage 1: No significant hair loss or recession of the hairline.

Stage 2: There is a slight recession of the hairline around the temples. This is also known as an adult or mature hairline.

Stage 3: The first signs of clinically significant balding appear. The hairline becomes deeply recessed at both temples, resembling an M, U, or V shape. The recessed spots are completely bare or sparsely covered in hair.

Stage 3 – vertex: The hairline stays at stage 2 or 3, but there is significant hair loss on the top of the scalp (the vertex).

Stage 4: The hairline recession is more severe than in stage 2 or 3, and there is sparse hair or no hair on the vertex. The two areas of hair loss are separated by a band of hair that connects to the hair remaining on the sides of the scalp.

Stage 5: The two areas of hair loss are larger than in stage IV. They are still separated, but the band of hair between them is narrower and sparser.

Stage 6: The balding areas at the temples join with the balding area at the vertex. The band of hair across the top of the head is gone or sparse.

Stage 7: The most severe stage of hair loss, only a band of hair going around the sides of the head remains. This hair is usually not dense and may be fine.

For women, the Ludwig scale is most commonly used (Figure 10.3):

Grade 1: Perceptible thinning of the hair on the crown, limited in the front by a line situated 1–3 cm behind the frontal hair line.

Grade 2: Pronounced rarefaction of the hair on the crown within the area seen in Grade 1.

Grade 3: Full baldness (total denudation) within the area seen in Grades 1 and 2.

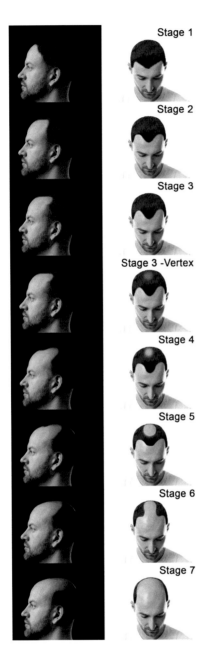

FIGURE 10.2   The Norwood classification for hair loss in men. (Based on Norwood OT. Male pattern baldness: Classification and incidence. *South Med J* 1975;68:1359–65.)

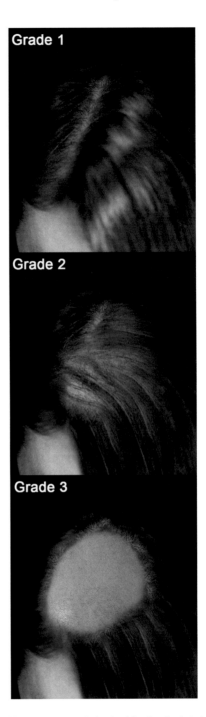

FIGURE 10.3   The Ludwig classification for hair loss in women. (Based on Ludwig E. Classification of the types of androgenetic alopecia [common baldness] occurring in the female sex. *Br J Dermatol.* 1977;97:247–54.)

Treatment Options

Treatments for hair thinning and hair loss can be divided into three broad categories: oral and topical solutions, minimally invasive treatments, and camouflage and surgical interventions. The treatments discussed below can be combined across all categories depending on the presentation of the patient to achieve personalised aesthetic goals.

Oral and Topical Solutions

Suitable for Those Who

- *Have very early signs of hair thinning and hair loss*
- *Have viable hair follicles*
- *Would like to prevent further hair loss*
- *Would like to manage hair loss without more invasive measures*

Minoxidil

Minoxidil was originally introduced as an antihypertensive drug [3]. However, a topical formulation was developed due to its common adverse effect, hypertrichosis. FDA-approved for use in men and women, minoxidil is one of the main over-the-counter treatments for androgenic alopecia, female pattern hair loss, and various off-license treatments for other hair loss and hair thinning conditions [4]. Two percent or 5% minoxidil solution are readily available and, in some patients, application to the scalp can help slow down the progression of alopecia and partially restore hair growth [3, 4]. However, the benefit is only maintained for as long as the treatment is used [3]. Furthermore, minoxidil has been known to cause irritation or allergic reactions in some patients [3].

Side Effects

- Severe scalp irritation
- Palpitations
- Unwanted facial hair growth
- Flushing (warmth, redness, or tingly feeling)
- Dizziness or light-headedness

Finasteride

Finasteride is another FDA-approved medication to treat male pattern hair loss (androgenic alopecia) [5, 6]. It is a 5α-reductase inhibitor that works by reducing the production of dihydrotestosterone (DHT) [5, 6]. DHT is responsible for the miniaturisation of hair follicles in men, reducing their ability to support a healthy head of hair. Finasteride has been shown to reduce hair loss by approximately 30% within 6 months of use with most result seen in the crown area [5]. This is due to its ability to maintain or increase the number of healthy hair follicles by inhibiting and reversing miniaturisation of hair follicles [5, 6]. However, the effectiveness only persists for as long as the drug is taken [6, 7]. Recognised side effects include decreased libido and erectile dysfunction [6, 7]. Any beneficial effects on hair growth will be lost within 6–12 months of discontinuing treatment [7]. The use of finasteride in women has been a subject of debate for years, with some studies showing no significant improvement compared to placebo group [8]. However, recent studies have shown increased hair thickness and arrested hair loss in women suffering from angrogenic alopecia who had been taking daily finasteride for 3 years [8]. The use of topical finasteride has also been studied in recent years amongst men and women with promising preliminary results; significant decrease in scalp and plasma DHT was observed without changes in serum testosterone (and therefore less side effects compared to oral administration) [9].

Side Effects

- Low libido
- Impotence
- Trouble having an orgasm
- Dizziness
- Skin rash
- Headache
- Abnormal ejaculation

Minimally Invasive Treatments

Suitable for Those Who

- *Have early to late signs of hair thinning and hair loss*
- *Have viable hair follicles*
- *Would like to restore hair growth*
- *Would like to prevent further hair loss*

Platelet-Rich Plasma (PRP)

Hair restoration is one of the most highly supported indications for platelet-rich plasma (PRP) in aesthetic medicine. This treatment involves initial venipuncture to obtain 10–30 ml of whole blood in blood collection tubes containing an anticoagulant agent. The whole blood sample is then placed into a centrifuge, which separates the blood into three distinct layers: red blood cells, platelet-poor plasma, and PRP. The harvested PRP is then injected into the scalp at a depth of approximately 4 mm. The growth factors released by the platelets are thought to help improve the quality and number of hair produced by active hair follicles [10]. Vascular endothelial growth factor (VEGF) and platelet-derived growth factor (PDGF) are known to be pro-angiogenesis, which would help improve the microcirculation of the target area. The growth factors released are also thought to help with stem cell activation and reduction of hair follicle inflammation (which reduces the number and quality of hair produced) [10, 11]. PRP is often used to treat androgenic alopecia, and treatment protocols vary as follows [10]:

a. PRP injections alone (injected every 2–3 weeks for 12 weeks)
b. PRP injections with dalteparin and protamine microparticles (injected every 2–3 weeks for 12 weeks)
c. PRP injections with progesterone (injected every 4 weeks for 24 weeks, then every 8–12 weeks indefinitely)
d. PRP injections with CD34+ cells (injected every 3 months)

Injections of PRP alone, and when combined with dalteparin and protamine, have shown to increase mean hair numbers post-treatment with significant increases in collagen, fibroblasts, and angiogenesis around hair follicles [12]. Greater increase in hair diameter was also observed in those treated with the combination of PRP, dalteparin, and protamine [13]. PRP administered with progesterone has the additional benefit of inhibiting 5-α reductase, resulting in the inhibition of DHT production and promotion of hair growth [10]. An increase in hair count, thickness, density, and cosmetic appearance has been reported in patients treated with the combination of PRP with CD34+ cells [10].

Complications

- Haematoma (needle trauma)
- Oedema (needle trauma)

- Erythema (needle trauma)
- Infection (lack of aseptic technique)

Growth Factor Induced Therapy (GFIT)

Growth factors are proteins that bind to receptors on cell membrane surface with the primary function of activating cellular activities. Acting as chemical messengers between cells, they play a role in cell proliferation, and their use has been reported to improve hair regrowth. Several therapeutic strategies have been suggested, including regeneration of hair follicles and reversing the pathological mechanisms that contribute to hair loss [14].

Human-derived growth factors obtained from a genetically modified fibroblast cell line have been used widely in the field of aesthetics for hair restoration and is approved by the FDA (AQ Skin Solutions). The cells are grown in enriched media for pure growth factor production; the growth factors, cytokines, interleukins, and other peptides produced by fibroblasts are then harvested and purified from the cell cultures. The active ingredients used in growth factor induced therapy (GFIT) treatment include:

a. Transforming growth factors (beta 1, 2, and 3), which help facilitate cell chemotaxis, inhibit matrix degradation, and stimulate glycosaminoglycan production

b. Granulocyte-macrophage colony-stimulating factor, which improves leukocyte function, activates neutrophils, eosinophils, and monocytes, and stimulates proliferation and differentiation of hematopoietic cell lines

c. Interleukins (IL-3, 6, 7, and 8), which help regulate cell homeostasis and function as anti-inflammatory agents

For those who do not respond to PRP or are deemed unsuitable (e.g. smokers), GFIT may be a more suitable option. This treatment involves delivering the highly concentrated serum to the target area via microneedling (0.8 mm). Microneedling performed with growth factors and active ingredients has shown some promising results on the improvement of hair growth [15]. Usually 10 weekly sessions are required, with a 2-week break after the 5th session. GFIT is safe to be repeated according to the progress of the patient.

Complications

- Oedema (microneedle trauma)
- Erythema (microneedle trauma)
- Infection (lack of aseptic technique)

Camouflage and Surgical Interventions

Suitable for Those Who

- *Have late signs of hair thinning and hair loss*
- *Have large areas of baldness*
- *Have failed to respond to other treatment modalities*
- *Do not have viable hair follicles in affected area*
- *Have viable hair follicles in surrounding areas*
- *Would like to have rapid results with a bigger difference after treatment*

Scalp Micropigmentation (SMP)

SMP is a form of medical tattooing where tiny dots are placed on the scalp simulating hair follicles. The medical grade ink used in this procedure (manufactured with scalp anatomy and physiology in mind) is placed in the superficial dermis, and results are expected to last between 3 and 7 years (typically 5 years on average) [16]. The depth of pigment implantation is key to a successful SMP procedure. If the ink is placed too deep, it will migrate leading to a solid unnatural look. On the other hand, if the ink placement is too superficial, the result will fade in a matter of weeks.

Careful fading is usually created towards the hairline and into any existing hair to create a seamless join or finish. The longevity of results is dependent on lifestyle factors and sun exposure – those with unhealthier lifestyle habits or prolonged exposure to the sun tend to have shorter duration of results. The treatment is carried out over three to four separate sittings, allowing the ink to settle after each session [16]. Results can be seen immediately; however, a completed treatment would take approximately 6 weeks. Each sitting can last from 30 to 60 minutes for a small patch of hair loss or a small scar, to several hours for an entire scalp treatment [16, 17]. SMP is ideal for both men and women at any stage of hair loss and is a viable option for an array of conditions, for example androgenetic alopecia and central centrifugal cicatricial alopecia (CCCA) which is often referred to as scarring alopecia.

SMP is also used to camouflage surgical or trauma scarring such as a follicular unit transplantation (FUT) strip scar following a hair transplant, a burn or an injury [17]. SMP can also be effective in combination with other hair restoration treatments where the illusion of density completes the treatment. For patients who are unsuitable for other restoration treatments, e.g. follicular unit extraction (FUE) procedure, SMP can be used as an ideal alternative [16, 17]. In male patients, a completed SMP treatment can provide the illusion of a full head of hair shaved to a buzz cut by choice, or to blend a thinning area. For female patients, SMP can cover areas of bare scalp, receding hair lines or exaggerated partings due to female pattern hair loss.

Complications

- Haematoma (needle trauma)
- Oedema (needle trauma)
- Erythema (needle trauma)
- Infection (lack of aseptic technique)
- Hypersensitivity or allergic reaction to dye
- Unnatural results (due to incorrect depth of ink placement)

Hair Transplant

There are two harvesting methods for hair transplantation, FUT and FUE. While they both share the same goal of moving healthy hair follicles from one area (donor site) to another (recipient site), the way hair follicles are harvested is vastly different.

First described in 1959, FUT has opened the way to hair transplantation and the field of hair replacement has been evolving continuously since [18]. Sometimes referred to as a 'strip' procedure, FUT involves removing a small strip of hair-bearing skin from the donor site. Under high powered microscopes, the strip is then dissected into individual follicular units, and each graft is then transplanted individually into the recipient site [18]. The defect created through the harvesting process is usually closed with stitches or staples, resulting in a thin linear scar. FUT allows for a large number of follicles or grafts to be harvested safely in a single setting and provides the ability for the patient to undergo more surgeries at a later date if necessary [18]. The procedure also boasts a consistently high growth yield with 95–98% successful growth rate [18]. However, the procedure may not be suitable for patients with tight scalps and a permanent linear scar is left behind.

FUE utilises small punches of 0.8–1 mm in diameter to extract follicular units [19]. As each follicular unit is extracted one-by-one, FUE is a more laborious, time-consuming procedure that depends highly on the skill of the surgeon; the number of grafts that can be harvested in one sitting is also less when compared to FUT [19]. After extraction, each follicle is separated from scalp tissue with the help of forceps, before being examined under a microscope and implanted into the recipient site. The stripping of hair follicles may result in poorer graft quality, and hence the results may be less consistent compared to FUT [20]. In each donor site, the small hole created is left open to heal into a dot scar. The benefits of

FUE include the ability to harvest from patients with tight scalps, higher level of patient comfort as well as small and barely visible scars [20].

Complications

- Scarring (especially at donor site)
- Haematoma (surgical trauma)
- Oedema (surgical trauma)
- Erythema (surgical trauma)
- Infection (lack of aseptic technique)
- Graft rejection (failure of graft to grow at recipient site)
- Delayed wound healing (due to underlying medical conditions such as diabetes)
- Suture extrusion (rare complication)
- Persistent pain – neuralgia, neuroma, and hypesthesia (due to deep incisions)

Case Study 10.1

Patient Age: 32
  Sex: Female

Presenting Concern

- Severe scarring alopecia

Treatment Plan

- SMP (three sessions)

Result

- Illusion of dense hair, shaved to a buzz cut by choice. See Figure 10.4.

Case Study 10.2 (Courtesy of Ms. Kelly Morrell)

Patient Age: 27
  Sex: Male

Presenting Concern

- Scarring due to unsuccessful FUE procedure. Although a second FUE was possible and offered to the patient, he remained traumatised and could not contemplate more surgery.

Grading (before)

- III (Norwood scale)

Treatment Plan

- SMP (after photo taken after one session)

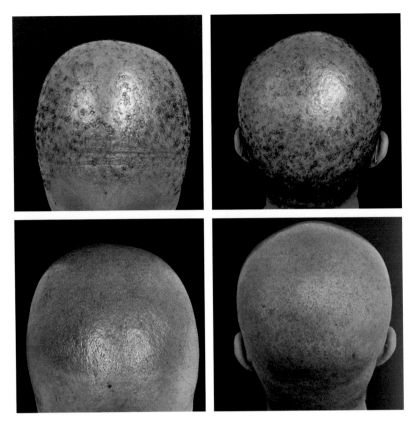

FIGURE 10.4 Top row: Before SMP, front view (left), and back view (right). Bottom row: After SMP, front view (left), and back view (right).

Grading (after)

- I (Norwood scale)

Result

- Illusion of active follicles in scarred areas, and dense hair shaved to a buzz cut by choice. See Figure 10.5.

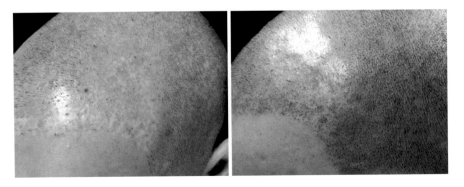

FIGURE 10.5 Hairline in the left frontal and temporal region before (left) and after (right) SMP.

Case Study 10.3

Patient Age: 26
  Sex: Female

Presenting Concern

- Hair thinning, even after hair transplant. Previously tried minoxidil and oral supplements without satisfactory outcome.

Grading (before)

- II (Ludwig scale)

Treatment Plan

- Hair restoration with GFIT from AQ Skin Solutions (10 sessions)

Grading (after)

- I (Ludwig scale)

Result

- Improved hair thickness and quality of hair. Results continued to improve beyond treatment period. See Figure 10.6.

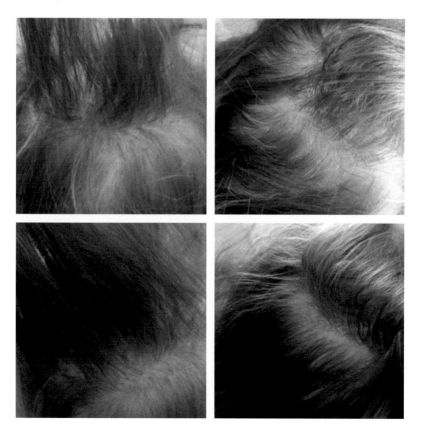

FIGURE 10.6   Density of hair in the crown area before (top row) and after (bottom row) 10 sessions of GFIT treatment.

Case Study 10.4

Patient Age: 29
  Sex: Male

Presenting Concern

- *Androgenic* alopecia: Patient was reluctant to try minoxidil or finasteride.

Grading (before)

- IV (Norwood scale)

Treatment Plan

- Hair restoration with GFIT from AQ Skin Solutions (ten sessions)

Grading (after)

- III Vertex (Norwood scale)

Result

- Improved hair density and hairline restoration. Results continued to improve beyond treatment period. See Figure 10.7.

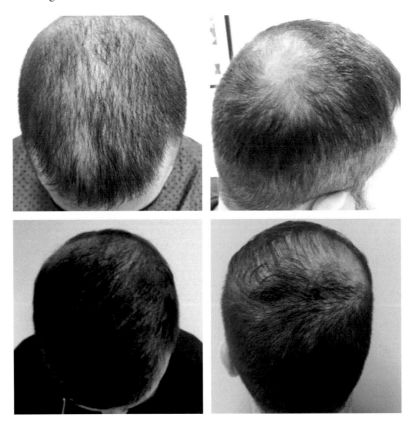

FIGURE 10.7   Density of hair before (top row) and after (bottom row) 10 sessions of GFIT treatment.

REFERENCES

1. Phillips TG, Slomiany WP, Allison R, "Hair loss: Common causes and treatment," *American Family Physician*, vol. 96, no. 6, pp. 371–378, 2017.
2. Vañó-Galván S, "Frequency of the types of alopecia at twenty-two specialist hair clinics: A multicenter study," *Skin Appendage Disorders*, vol. 5, no. 5, pp. 309–315, 2019.
3. Suchonwanit P, Thammarucha A, Leerunyakul K, "Minoxidil and its use in hair disorders: A review," *Drug Design, Development and Therapy*, vol. 9, no. 13, pp. 2777–2786, 2019.
4. Gupta AK, Foley KA, "5% Minoxidil: Treatment for female pattern hair loss," *Skin Therapy Letter*, vol. 9, no. 6, pp. 5–7, 2014.
5. Mysore V, Shashikumar BM, "Guidelines on the use of finasteride in androgenetic alopecia," *Indian Journal of Dermatology, Venereology and Leprology*, vol. 82, no. 2, pp. 128–134, 2016.
6. Motofei IG, Rowland DL, Tampa M, et al. "Finasteride and androgenic alopecia; from therapeutic options to medical implications," *Journal of Dermatological Treatment*, vol. 31, no. 4, pp. 415–421, 2020.
7. Carreño-Orellana N, Moll-Manzur C, Carrasco-Zuber JE, Álvarez-Véliz S, Berroeta-Mauriziano D, Porras-Kusmanic N, "Finasteride adverse effects: An update," *Revista Medica de Chile*, vol. 144, no. 12, pp. 1584–1590, 2016.
8. Hu AC, Chapman LW, Mesinkovska NA, "The efficacy and use of finasteride in women: A systematic review," *International Journal of Dermatology*, vol. 58, no. 7, pp. 759–776, 2019.
9. Lee SW, Juhasz M, Mobasher P, Ekelem C, Mesinkovska NA, "A systematic review of topical finasteride in the treatment of androgenetic alopecia in men and women," *Journal of Drugs in Dermatology*, vol. 17, no. 4, pp. 457–463, 2018.
10. Emer J, "Platelet-rich plasma (PRP): Current applications in dermatology," *Skin Therapy Letter*, vol. 24, no. 5, pp. 1–6, 2019.
11. Rodrigues BL, Montalvão SAL, Cancela RBB, "Treatment of male pattern alopecia with platelet-rich plasma: A double-blind controlled study with analysis of platelet number and growth factor levels," *Journal of the American Academy of Dermatology*, vol. 80, no. 3, pp. 694–700, 2019.
12. Leo MS, Kumar AS, Kirit R, Konathan R, Sivamani RK, "Systematic review of the use of platelet-rich for aesthetic dermatology," *Journal of Cosmetic Dermatology*, vol. 14, no. 4, pp. 315–323, 2015.
13. Takikawa M, Nakamura S, Nakamura S, et al. "Enhanced effect of platelet rich plasma containing a new carrier on hair growth," *Dermatologic Surgery*, vol. 37, no. 12, pp. 1721–1729, 2011.
14. Gentile P, Garcovich S, "Advances in regenerative stem cell therapy in androgenic alopecia and hair loss: Wnt pathway, growth-factor, and mesenchymal stem cell signaling impact analysis on cell growth and hair follicle development," *Cells*, vol. 8, no. 5, p. 466, 2019.
15. Fertig RM, Gamret AC, Cervantes J, Tosti A, "Microneedling for the treatment of hair loss?," *Journal of the European Academy of Dermatology and Venereology*, vol. 32, no. 4, pp. 564–569, 2018.
16. Rassman WR, Pak JP, Kim J, "Scalp micropigmentation: A useful treatment for hair loss," *Facial Plastic Surgery Clinics of North America*, vol. 21, no. 3, pp. 497–503, 2013.
17. Rassman WR, Pak JP, Kim J, Estrin NF, "Scalp micropigmentation: A concealer for hair and scalp deformities," *The Journal of Clinical and Aesthetic Dermatology*, vol. 8, no. 3, pp. 35–42, 2015.
18. Jiménez-Acosta F, Ponce I, "Follicular unit hair transplantation: Current technique," *Actas Dermosifiliográficas*, vol. 101, no. 4, pp. 291–306, 2010.
19. Sharma R, Ranjan A, "Follicular unit extraction (FUE) hair transplant: Curves ahead," *Journal of Maxillofacial and Oral Surgery*, vol. 18, no. 4, pp. 509–517, 2019.
20. Kerure AS, Patwardhan N, "Complications in hair transplantation," *Journal of Cutaneous and Aesthetic Surgery*, vol. 11, no. 1, pp. 182–189, 2018.

11

Balancing Non-Surgical and Surgical Clinical Approaches

Mehmet Veli Karaaltin, Adnan Erdem, and Vincent Wong

CONTENTS

Clinical approach to facial rejuvenation requires a perception of integrity and customised analysis for each individual patient. As discussed in Chapter 1, patient selection is one of the key factors to a successful cosmetic procedure – most patients want to look refreshed, and a thorough consultation will determine the appropriate treatment plan. Another vital factor is to understand the limitations of non-surgical options and have a good understanding of what surgical procedures have to offer. Whilst many procedures are best performed non-surgically, there are certain goals or outcomes that can only be realised by surgery.

The face and neck areas are amongst the most complex regions of the human body, due to the complicated interplay between different structures (bones, ligaments, muscles, fat, and skin). Ageing occurs in all facial structures, but the onset and the speed of age-related changes differ between each specific structure, between each individual, between different ethnic groups as well as genetic background. Therefore, knowledge of age-related anatomy is crucial when trying to restore a youthful face.

In this chapter, we will explore how both surgical and non-surgical approaches can help patients achieve their personalised aesthetic goals, especially in complex cases where more than one treatment modality is required. Although some crossovers exist between what surgical and non-surgical techniques can achieve, there is still a wide variation in indications for different treatment modalities. A combined, holistic treatment approach may produce better aesthetic outcomes in these patients and avoid unnatural-looking results. Furthermore, non-surgical treatments can also be used to maintain results obtained from surgery. The unique clinical cases presented in this chapter will highlight the importance of having a customised algorithm for each patient with multiple procedures (both surgical and non-surgical) included in the treatment plan, pushing facial rejuvenation to a new level in the concept of 'thinking outside the box'.

Review of Facial Ageing

Ageing Skin

Skin is a complex organ covering the entire surface of the body. Aged skin is characterised by the appearance of wrinkles, hypermelanosis, increased laxity, and loss of volume. These changes occur under the influence of intrinsic and extrinsic factors. Therefore, knowledge of skin histology and physiology, as discussed in Chapter 2, will provide a deeper understanding of cutaneous changes associated with chronological and photo-ageing, which will, in turn, help physicians achieve better cosmetic and functional outcomes [1].

Ageing of Muscles, Ligaments, and Fat Compartments

The superficial muscular-aponeurotic system (SMAS) is a layer of organised fibrous network composed of muscle fibres, fascia, fat as well as a fibromuscular layer. With such unique composition and connection to facial muscles and the skin, it helps to coordinate muscular contractions of the face and provides a functional role of movement for facial expression. The facial retaining ligaments act as anchor points to tether the skin and underlying layers to the facial skeleton [1–3]. With time, deep facial structures tend to sag and hood over these fixing points, creating folds and ptoses which exacerbates the appearance of an aged face. There are multiple fat compartments in the face and neck [4, 5], which typically lose volume and migrate with age. Facial muscles also develop tone over time, which can lead to shortening, weakening, and straightening.

Ageing of the Facial Skeleton

The skeletal structure of the face creates the foundation for the soft tissue covering it. However, the facial skeleton undergoes morphological changes with increasing age, especially around the orbit (eye socket tends to become wider and larger with age). The composition, robustness as well as volume also start to decline with time, hence affecting the face in a negative way [1–5].

Assessment Algorithm for a Personalised Holistic Clinical Approach

The decision-making process when it comes to facial aesthetics is not a straightforward one and is often influenced by physician factors (e.g. knowledge, skills, range of services) and patient factors (e.g. lifestyle, budget, downtime, expectations). However, the treatment plan proposed to the patient should be guided by scientific foundations built on professional experience, physical examination, patient status as well as an honest and thorough consultation prior to the procedure.

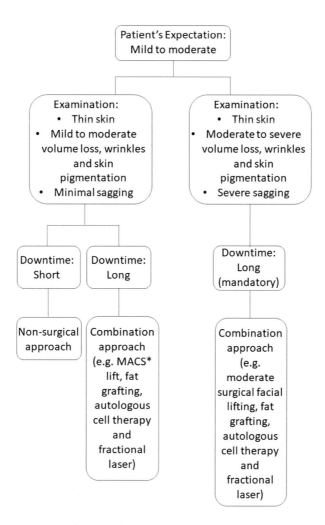

FIGURE 11.1   Algorithm suggested for patients with mild to moderate outcome expectations. (Courtesy of Prof. Mehmet Veli Karaaltin and Mr. Adnan Erdem.)

The algorithms in Figures 11.1 and 11.2 have been developed through years of clinical experience and patient interactions and could be a useful guide in clinical practice to meet patients' expectations. It highlights the indications for surgical and non-surgical procedures, and most importantly, where both modalities can work in synergy.

General Considerations

Autologous Fat or Dermal Fillers?

Volume loss is a common presentation of chronological ageing, and the restoration of lost volume plays a huge role in restoring a youthful visage. There are two options when it comes to facial volumisation: dermal fillers and autologous fat transfer. Although the injection techniques used for extracted fat tissue are hugely similar to dermal fillers, there are advantages and disadvantages to both, making

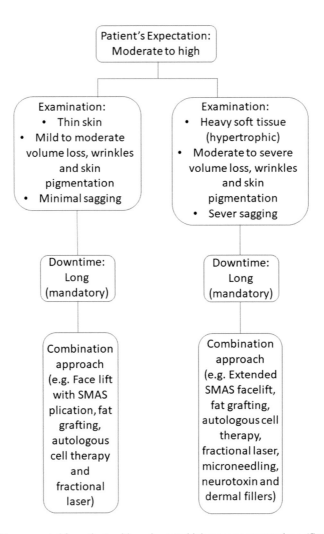

FIGURE 11.2   Algorithm suggested for patients with moderate to high outcome expectations. (Courtesy of Prof. Mehmet Veli Karaaltin and Mr. Adnan Erdem.) *Note.* SMAS = Superficial muscular-aponeurotic system.

it difficult to decide which is best for the patients. Fat injections tend to have longer-lasting result; however, approximately 50% of the transferred fat will disappear over a few months due to failure to obtain a blood supply in the recipient side. As discussed in previous chapters, this can be reduced by mixing the fat tissue with platelet-rich plasma (PRP) or autologous cell therapy (e.g. adipose-derived stromal vascular fraction cells). As the extraction process of the fat is a surgical procedure (especially in cases where a large amount of fat is required), it has a longer recovery time and will usually cost more to the patient. Dermal fillers on the other hand are readily available, with shorter recovery time. However, the effects of dermal filler injections are short-lived and if a large amount of volume is required, dermal fillers may be more expensive than autologous fat transfer. There is usually a 'tipping point' where one option is more desirable; this could be influenced by many factors such as volume required, financial issues, the desire to use autologous tissue, and the magnitude of result desired. In some cases, both treatments may also be part of the treatment plan – for example, some patients may consider having fat transfer as a starting point, followed by subsequent injections of dermal fillers to achieve the desired look.

Facial Rejuvenation with Fat Compartment Shifting and Enhancement

Several studies have shown the chronological changes to the fat compartments of the face and neck and their clinical implications for facial rejuvenation [4, 5]. Some fat compartments undergo hypertrophy whilst others lose volume over time – this varies between individuals and ethnic backgrounds. This volume 'drift' leads to a 'sheared' effect – the face and neck lose definition and smoothness over time, contributing to a saggy appearance. The concept of fat compartment shifting and enhancement involves volume enhancement and reduction in the appropriate areas, as well as soft-tissue repositioning. The use of adipose-derived stromal vascular fraction cells and PRP further enhances the effect of this powerful treatment concept, as demonstrated in the following case studies [6].

Clinical Case 11.1

A 41-year-old female patient who had bariatric surgery 2 years ago suffered from accelerated skin and facial soft-tissue sagging with lipoatrophy in the midfacial region. Due to occupational reasons, she rejected invasive procedures. A fat compartment shifting with stromal vascular fraction treatment was indicated. In the procedure, volume enhancement was indicated in the midface, lateral zygoma, premental fat, retro orbicularis oculi fat (ROOF), superficial orbicularis oculi fat (SOOF), supraorbital fat, frontal forehead fat compartment, marginal mandibular rim fat, and nasolabial fold. The volume enhancement was performed with structural fat grafting combined with stromal vascular fraction cells prepared with enzymatic separation (Biotrend Inc., Beauty Cell CE. Istanbul, Turkey). Volume reduction was performed in the submental fat compartment, subplatysmal fat compartment, and the inferior jowl fat compartment. See Figures 11.3 and 11.4.

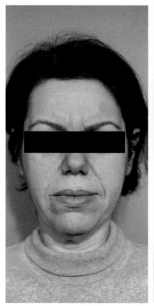 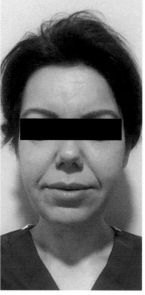

FIGURE 11.3 Frontal view of patient before (left) and after (right) treatment. (Courtesy of Prof. Mehmet Veli Karaaltin and Mr. Adnan Erdem.)

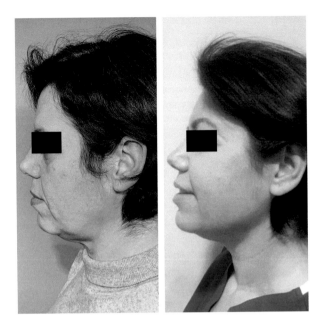

FIGURE 11.4   Profile view of patient before (left) and after (right) treatment. (Courtesy of Prof. Mehmet Veli Karaaltin and Mr. Adnan Erdem.)

Clinical Case 11.2

A 43-year-old female patient, suffering from double chin deformity and loss of jawline definition. A premental fat enhancement with structural and nano-fat grafting, along with liposuction to the submental, subplatysmal and jowl regions, was performed. A satisfactory rejuvenation with moderate lifting effect was achieved. See Figure 11.5.

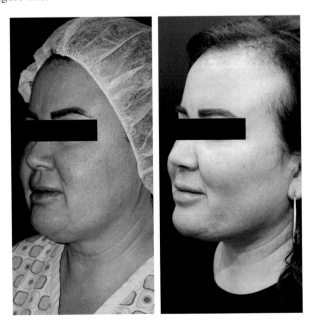

FIGURE 11.5   Forty-five-degree side view of patient before (left) and after (right) treatment. (Courtesy of Prof. Mehmet Veli Karaaltin and Mr. Adnan Erdem.)

Clinical Case 11.3

A 68-year-old patient with signs of facial ageing had a total parotidectomy due to malignancy, with postoperative radiotherapy for 5 years pre-treatment. The patient had a single structural fat injection to the parotid nest in order to treat Frey's syndrome. A face lift procedure was avoided due to the high risk of facial nerve injury. Volume reduction from the submental and jowl areas as well as fat grafting to the midface, preorbital, frontal, lateral zygomatic, marginal mandibular and mental regions were performed. See Figure 11.6.

Understanding the Limits and Boundaries in Volumising Methods

One of most common mistakes in autologous structural fat grafting or non-invasive volume enhancing procedures with dermal fillers is the indefinite selection of treatment areas, leading to an over-filled or 'done' look. The face and neck comprise of ten distinct compartments, each encapsulated with ligaments and separated by septum [4]. It is therefore crucial to assess the condition of each individual compartment as well as the relationship with neighbouring compartments and any overlapping areas. The volumising procedure should only be performed in specific areas where volume enhancement is required in order to achieve maximum yield whilst respecting facial proportions, balance, and harmony. Other factors of ageing (e.g. cutaneous, muscle, and bone changes) should also be considered.

Volumising Methods Should Compensate and Revert the Skeletal Changes through Age

Skeletal atrophy as well as dentition problems exacerbates the appearance of ageing signs. Several studies have shown that the maxillary projection and its piriform angle decrease with age. As the underlying maxilla provides the essential projection around the nose, these bony changes are likely to contribute to the appearance of mid-face ageing, such as prominent nasolabial folds, facial hollowing, loss of dentition,

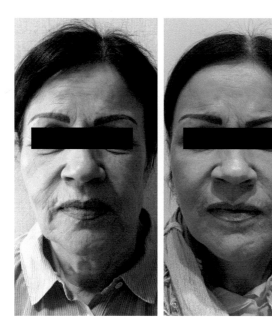

FIGURE 11.6 Frontal view of patient before (left) and after (right) treatment. (Courtesy of Prof. Mehmet Veli Karaaltin and Mr. Adnan Erdem.)

and the senile nose [7]. The following key points should be taken into consideration when performing facial rejuvenation (either surgical or non-surgical):

1. Ageing of the periorbital region includes skeletal changes such as skeletal retrusion and widening of the orbit in the superomedial and inferolateral aspects (as discussed in Chapter 4).
2. A parallel retrusion rate occurs in the maxillary and zygomatic regions.
3. As we age, the nose elongates, with decreased nasal tip projection and posterior displacement of nasal alae [7].
4. The bigonial distance and ramus width show no significant chronological changes; however, the height and length of the mandible decreases [8]
5. The Negative Vector

As discussed in Chapter 4, a negative vector exists when the most anterior globe portion protrudes past the malar eminence. Indeed, the negative vector of the face is another challenging condition in facial rejuvenation treatment. A prominent globe or atrophy of the malar area results in a negative vector in the periorbital area – any aesthetic procedures performed without first correcting the negative vector may worsen the patient's appearance [9]. In this group of patients, the bone structures, lower eyelid, malar fat compartments and related ligaments must be assessed and addressed individually [9].

The Benjamin Button Effect

Inspired by the popular motion picture, the Benjamin Button effect is used to describe the goal of achieving a clearly younger, more attractive, yet natural-looking appearance utilising minimally invasive therapies [10]. The same concept can also be applied when it comes to combining surgical and non-surgical modalities; non-surgical treatments can be utilised after an invasive face lift procedure to enhance the outcome and longevity of results. See Figures 11.7 and 11.8.

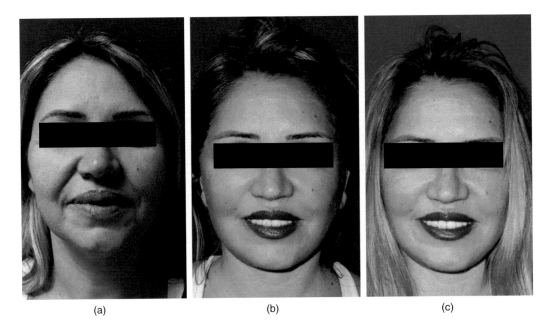

(a)   (b)   (c)

FIGURE 11.7 Frontal view of a 50-year-old female patient who had an extended high SMAS face lift procedure: (a) before the procedure; (b) 2 years after the procedure at age 52 (with at-home treatments described above, regular visits for non-surgical treatments and use of medical-grade skincare products); (c) 6 years after the initial procedure, at age 56. (Courtesy of Prof. Mehmet Veli Karaaltin and Mr. Adnan Erdem.)

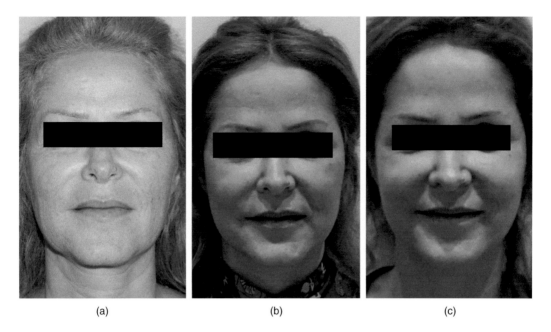

(a)	(b)	(c)

FIGURE 11.8 Frontal view of a 57-year-old female patient who had an extended high SMAS face lift procedure: (a) before the procedure; (b) 2 years after the procedure, at age 59 (with at-home treatments described above, regular visits for non-surgical treatments and use of medical-grade skinacre products); (c) 4 years after the initial procedure, at age 61. (Courtesy of Prof. Mehmet Veli Karaaltin and Mr. Adnan Erdem.)

Typically, patients who underwent cosmetic surgery would be encouraged to use topical liposomal epidermal growth factor with self-microneedling (1 mm) for 10 minutes for 1 month [6, 11, 12]. This at-home regime is repeated annually, whilst maintaining regular clinic visits for non-surgical treatments such as neurotoxin injections and skin resurfacing treatments, as well as the continuous use of medical-grade skincare products.

Treating Facial Traumas with Anti-Ageing Concepts, Regenerative Medicine, and Face Lifting

Certain conditions, such as facial trauma due to road traffic accidents and other assaults, can cause drastic changes that might lead to an accelerated ageing process which does not correlate to the patient's actual age. A combination of plastic surgery, regenerative medicine, and anti-ageing treatments can help physicians obtain the best aesthetic outcome in such challenging cases.

The facial skin in most circumstances is directly affected by the trauma. Apart from surface irregularities and scarring, skin elasticity is also reduced, increasing the tendency to sag. This is due to physical changes as well as lipoatrophy. Furthermore, pigmentation and other topographical changes can also worsen the patient's appearance. All these parameters should be addressed meticulously when formulating a treatment plan. Combining surgical correction with non-surgical treatments (e.g. growth factor induced therapy, PRP and autologous cell therapy) can boost the regenerative capacity of the human body; this healing potential can have a huge impact on the patient's overall wellbeing and quality of life [13, 14]. See Figure 11.9.

Closing Lines

Our facial appearance is often seen as a reflection of our inner well-being. Indeed, they are often interlinked, and one can have a direct impact on the other. Regardless of the patient's history and presentation, each healthcare professional in the field of facial aesthetics has a duty to help patients match their

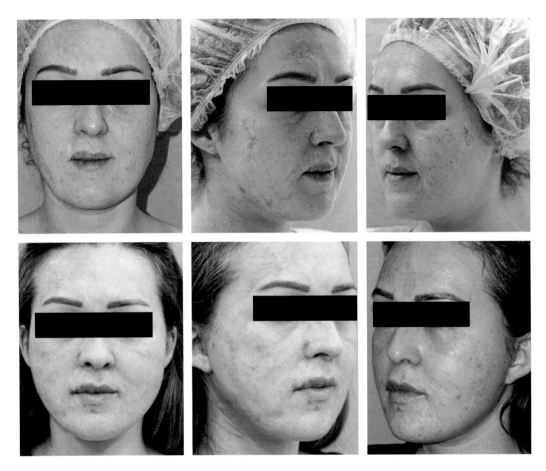

FIGURE 11.9 Frontal and quadrant views of a 27-year-old female patient who had corrective surgical facelift due to premature ageing (after a road traffic accident), combined with microdermabrasion, dermal micro-fat grafting, nano-fat grafting, epidermal growth factor injections (SP1-EGF, Bioceltran, South Korea) and epidermal cell suspension (ReCell Avita Medical Inc., UK). Photos in the top row were taken before surgery. Photos in the bottom row were taken 6 months after combination of treatments. (Courtesy of Prof. Mehmet Veli Karaaltin and Mr. Adnan Erdem.)

outer appearance with their truest inner identity. The final decision on which treatments we employ to fulfil this duty truly lies within our knowledge, skill set, and our understanding and awareness of what treatment options are available and what they can achieve.

REFERENCES

1. Alghoul M, Codner MA, "Retaining ligaments of the face: Review of anatomy and clinical applications," *Aesthetic Surgery Journal*, vol. 33, no. 6, pp. 769–82, 2013.
2. Charafeddine AH, Drake R, McBride J, Zins JE, "Facelift: History and anatomy," *Clinics in Plastic Surgery*, vol. 46, no. 4, pp. 505–513, 2019.
3. Seo YS, Song JK, Oh TS, Kwon SI, Tansatit T, Lee JH, "Review of the nomenclature of the retaining ligaments of the cheek: Frequently confused terminology," *Archives of Plastic Surgery*, vol. 44, no. 4, pp. 266–275, 2017.
4. Rohrich RJ, Pessa JE, "The fat compartments of the face: Anatomy and clinical implications for cosmetic surgery," *Plastic and Reconstructive Surgery*, vol. 119, no. 7, pp. 2219–2227, 2007.
5. Gassman AA, Pezeshk R, Scheuer JF 3rd, Sieber DA, Campbell CF, Rohrich RJ, "Anatomical and clinical implications of the deep and superficial fat compartments of the neck," *Plastic and Reconstructive Surgery*, vol. 140, no. 3, 405e–414e, 2017.

6. Charles-de-Sá L, Gontijo-de-Amorim NF, Maeda Takiya C, et al. "Antiaging treatment of the facial skin by fat graft and adipose-derived stem cells," *Plastic and Reconstructive Surgery*, vol. 135, no. 4, pp. 999–1009, 2015.

7. Paskhover B, Durand D, Kamen E, Gordon NA, "Patterns of change in facial skeletal aging," *JAMA Facial Plastic Surgery*, vol. 19, no. 5, pp. 413–417, 2017.

8. Mendelson B, Wong C-H, "Changes in the facial skeleton with aging: Implications and clinical applications in facial rejuvenation," *Aesthetic Plastic Surgery*, vol. 36, no. 4, pp. 753–760, 2012.

9. Mommaerts MY, "Definitive treatment of the negative vector orbit," *Journal of Cranio-Maxillofacial Surgery*, vol. 46, no. 7, pp. 1065–1068, 2018.

10. Waldorf HA, "Benjamin button effect: Recognizable rejuvenation," *Journal of Drugs in Dermatology*, vol. 16, no. 6, pp. s74–s76, 2017.

11. Harris AG, Naidoo C, Murrell DF, "Skin needling as a treatment for acne scarring: An up-to-date review of the literature," *International Journal of Women's Dermatology*, vol. 1, no. 2, pp. 77–81, 2015.

12. Ternullo S, Basnet P, Holsæter AM, Flaten GE, de Weerd L, Škalko-Basnet N, "Deformable liposomes for skin therapy with human epidermal growth factor: The effect of liposomal surface charge," *European Journal of Pharmaceutical Sciences*, vol. 125, pp. 163–171, 2018.

13. Sarangal R, Yadav S, Sakral A, Dogra S, "Noncultured epidermal-melanocyte cell suspension and dermal-fat grafting for the reconstruction of an irregular, atrophic, and depigmented forehead scar: An innovative approach," *Journal of Cosmetic Dermatology*, vol. 14, no. 4, pp. 332–335, 2015.

14. Tresoldi MM, Graziano A, Malovini A, Faga A, Nicoletti G, "The role of autologous dermal micrografts in regenerative surgery: A clinical experimental study," *Stem Cells International*, Sep. 8 2019, 9843407.

Index

Note: Locators in *italics* represent figures.

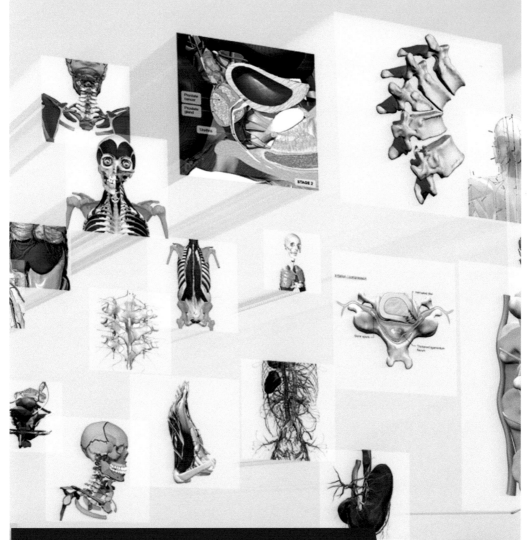